Psychiatric Emergencies in Pediatrics

AMAN U. KHAN, M.D.
Associate Professor of Pediatrics and Psychiatry
Northwestern University Medical School
Chicago, Illinois

YEAR BOOK MEDICAL PUBLISHERS, INC.
CHICAGO • LONDON

Library of Congress Cataloging in Publication Data

Khan, Aman U
Psychiatric emergencies in pediatrics.

Includes index.
1. Crisis intervention (Psychiatry). 2. Child psychiatry. 3. Psychiatric hospitals—Outpatient services. I. Title.
RJ504.4.K47 362.7'8'21 79–17978
ISBN 0–8151–5029–6

To my family (Jadine, Kamal, Aleisha and Jason),
whose support, affection and encouragement
allowed me to create and complete this book

Preface

IN THE LAST DECADE, hospitals have been forced to reexamine their outpatient services because of the increasing number of patients who have been using these facilities. In 1972, 95% of the hospitals in the United States reported more than 222 million outpatient visits. Of 7,105 hospitals with outpatient services, general hospitals provided 90% of the services and reported 213 million outpatient visits. The number of emergency room visits has increased at a faster rate than either hospital inpatient admissions or outpatient visits. The number of patient visits to emergency rooms tripled (increased by 40 million) during the 10-year period between 1962 and 72. Although separate data are not available for children and adolescents, it is estimated that at least 30% of these outpatient and emergency room visits are made by persons under 18 years of age.

This increase in utilization of outpatient services has also forced hospitals to employ full-time physicians to provide medical care in emergency rooms and other outpatient clinics. It is estimated that at least 10% of all hospital-based full-time physicians (approximately 2,500), as well as some 5,000 interns and residents, are providing full-time services in emergency rooms and other acute care clinics. In addition, a large number of nurses (approximately 40,000) are involved in these services, as are a growing number of medical social workers, psychologists and psychiatrists.

Data from emergency rooms and other acute care clinics indicate that clear-cut psychiatric diagnoses amount to about 2–5% of the total diagnostic categories. These figures are deceptive, however, and greatly underestimate the presence of psychiatric problems in emergency rooms. The low figures are attributable to the reluctance of physicians to make a psychiatric diagnosis and to the busy schedule of emergency rooms, which rarely permit the physician an opportunity to explore the emotional aspects of the medical problems he treats.

This book is designed to help physicians understand and manage the psychiatric problems commonly encountered in emergency rooms and acute care clinics. It treats the dynamics of these problems and provides step-by-step directions for their management.

Although some of the information contained in these pages may be found in various books and journal articles, this is the first book to describe these psychiatric problems in a practical and succinct manner for those professionals working in emergency rooms and acute care clinics. Several chapters contain original material drawn from long clinical experience in this field.

It is my hope that this book will serve as a handy reference for physicians, nurses, social workers, psychologists and psychiatrists working in emergency rooms and acute care clinics and that it will help to improve the psychiatric aspect of pediatric care.

I gratefully acknowledge the assistance provided by Joseph Cataio, who contributed considerably to the organizing, editing and proofreading of this book.

I would also like to thank Mrs. Irma Wallner and Ms. Cindy Lee, who were extremely helpful in the typing and preparation of this manuscript.

Contents

1/Hospitalism, Hospitalization and Day Care

HOSPITALISM has been defined as "a vitiated condition of the body due to long confinement in a hospital . . . the evil effect of institutional care of infants from an early age" (Spitz, 1945). This definition is very restricted, since there are few institutions today that provide long-term care to infants without attempting to meet their psychological needs. At present, most institutions caring for young children attempt to monitor and evaluate the psychological effects they have on their patients.

It is important to distinguish between hospitalism, a condition resulting from long-term hospitalization in infancy in an emotionally cold and sterile environment, and short-term hospitalization of children of all ages.

Day care centers for infants and children present yet another situation where children are separated from their parents and are cared for by persons who are initially strangers. These institutions, although rapidly increasing in number, have been the subject of much social debate regarding their possible adverse psychological effects on children.

The following section describes the historical events that led to the discovery of the phenomenon of hospitalism and to an understanding of the problems associated with separation and maternal deprivation.

Attachment

In the early part of this century, disastrous mortality rates brought institutional care of infants under severe attack. Chapin (1915a, b) enumerated 10 asylums in large American cities in which the death rate of infants admitted during their first year of life varied from 31.7% to 75%. In the same year, Knox (Chapin, 1915b) stated that in the child care institutions of Baltimore, 90% of the infants died by the end of their first year of institutionalization.

Conditions improved by the fourth and fifth decades. Bakwin (1942) reported a mortality rate of less than 10% for Bellevue Hospital in New York City. While these and similar results were being achieved both in this country and in Europe, physicians and administrators were faced with a new problem: they discovered that institutionalized children frequently developed subsequent psychiatric disturbances—delinquency, mental retardation and other psychiatric problems. The high mortality rate in preceding years had obscured these consequences. Now that the children survived, other drawbacks of institutionalization became apparent.

Several reports of the psychiatric consequences of institutional care of infants in their first year have appeared (Durfee and Wolf, 1933; Lowrey, 1940; Bender and Yarnell, 1941; Goldfarb, 1943). The psychological injury suffered by these infants was attributed to two primary factors—lack of stimulation and the absence of the infant's mother. It was emphasized that a home-reared infant always received more stimulation than a nursery-reared infant and that mothers provided more intensive stimulation than did nursing personnel. Those institutions in which mothers were available to care for their infants had lower infant mortality levels than institutions where only trained pediatric nurses were employed.

Spitz (1945) studied 164 children during their first year of life, of whom 130 were institutionalized and 34 home-reared. The institutions were categorized as "nursery" and "foundling homes." The nursery was in a penal institution where delinquent girls were sequestered. These girls delivered their babies in a nearby hospital and then cared for their children in the nursery of the penal institution, where they spent a great deal of time loving and cuddling their children under the supervision of the nursery staff. Foundling homes were very sterile, unstimulating medical environments with daily medical rounds and a nursing staff. The home-reared infants and nursery infants did significantly better than foundling home infants on all measures of development. In addition to developmental retardation, foundling home infants showed, from the third month on, an extreme susceptibility to all kinds of infection and illness.

Bowlby (1946), in a retrospective study, demonstrated that maternal deprivation was a common factor in the background of juvenile delinquents. More recent studies (Barry, 1949; Brown, 1961) support some of Bowlby's findings. Glueck and Glueck (1950) studied 500 persistently delinquent boys in their early teens. As a control, each delinquent boy was matched with a nondelinquent boy for age, intelligence, national origin and residence. They found that delinquent boys had significantly more losses in their childhood than had the children in the control group. The losses included parental death, divorce, separation, desertion and prolonged absence due to illness or imprisonment of the parents.

Some of the implications of Bowlby's work were accepted uncritically for many years and were interpreted to mean that any separation of the infant from the mother resulted in emotional deprivation. However, once the shock of his findings wore off, investigators began to ask more specific questions:

Why does the infant become so attached to his mother?

What is there in the mother-child relationship the deprivation of which caused such a disastrous effect?

The traditional interpretation of the close relationship between an infant and his mother assumed that the relationship was based on a conditioning process in which the mother, through association with such rewarding stimuli as food and warmth, became a rewarding stimulus herself in much the same way as the buzzer becomes a sign of food and a rewarding stimulus for dogs in a Pavlovian conditioning experiment. If the initial feeding experience was not rewarding, it was believed the infant would develop an unsatisfactory attachment to the mother.

This conditioning model of social learning has been refined by ethological experiments, especially those of Lorenz (1960) and Harlow (1962). These researchers contend that the attachment between infant and mother is not merely the result of the mother's attention to and care of the infant, but that there are additional factors inherent in the biologic nature of the infant that govern this attachment. Lorenz (1935) demonstrated that little ducklings soon after hatching will follow a moving object. Usually, this is the mother duck, but this following behavior can be elicited by any moving object, whether a wooden toy or a human being. This behavior is inherent in the newborn duckling and serves the purpose of species survival. It takes about 13 hours for the ducklings to become strongly attached to their first moving object, as demonstrated by the ducklings' avoiding any other moving object or expressing fear of other moving objects. In one of Harlow's experiments (1966), infant monkeys were fed from a milk bottle attached to a wire-mesh structure (wire-mesh mother). A similar structure was covered with terrycloth to provide soft, cuddly touch sensations (terrycloth mother). The infant monkeys spent most of their time cuddling the terrycloth mother and went to the wire-mesh mother only when hungry. The terrycloth mother seemed to make the infant monkey feel secure, as was inferred from an experiment in which a large wooden spider was placed in the room. The infant monkey looked frightened and ran to the terrycloth mother and not to the wire-mesh mother. These findings are interpreted as evidence of a strong inherent need in infant monkeys to cuddle (much like the ducklings' inherent need to follow). The infant monkey is born with a strong grasping reflex. In the natural environment of the jungle, the young monkey clings to the hairy undersurface of his mother for several months after birth. The infant monkey thus becomes attached to those objects that best simulate the tactile sensations received from clinging to the mother.

Apparently, each species has a special set of responses that can be brought forth at birth or very soon afterward. These responses are more complex than simple reflexes. They are elicited by the first appropriate stimulus that the environment provides, and the objects eliciting these responses usually become the objects of attachment for the young animal.

Animals who are deprived of appropriate attachment relationships with caring mothers of their species become isolated and do not learn to interact appropriately (socially or sexually) with other members of their species. The monkeys raised by terrycloth or wire-mesh mothers, although physically sound, would not play or mate well with other, normally raised, monkeys.

Ethological theories thus conclude that: (1) young animals are born with specific innate reactions, which (2) help them to survive and to develop an attachment to the appropriate members of their species, and (3) this attachment is considered essential for the later development of appropriate social and sexual behavior and relationships.

Are human infants born with such innate responses?

Bowlby (1946) has suggested that there are five such responses in the human infant: sucking, babbling, visual scanning, crying and smiling. They help the infant to survive, as well as promoting interaction between the infant and the mother, thus facilitating attachment. Sucking and crying have strong survival value, while babbling, visual scanning and smiling serve the purpose of promoting interaction with the mother.

The babbling that occurs during the first 6 weeks in human infants is an innate response. After the first 8 to 10 weeks, the environment seems to affect the frequency and variety of these sounds. Children raised in homes in which mother and child engage in reciprocal vocal play vocalize more and with greater variety than do infants from homes where such exchange is minimal.

There are two types of smiling responses: endogenous and exogenous. Endogenous smiling is present at birth. It is a spontaneous response associated with a specific EEG pattern within the rapid eye movement (REM) stage of sleep. It tends to occur in bursts and does not decline over successive REM periods. It is present even in microcephalic newborns and is more frequently displayed by premature infants. It is postulated that this form of smiling is mediated by brainstem structures and becomes inhibited by subsequent maturation of the cerebrum.

Exogenous smiling is not present at birth. It begins as an irregular response to external stimuli at the end of the first postnatal month. It promotes the interaction between the mother and the child, such interaction normally increasing the frequency of smiling.

Although there are normal variations in the frequency and strength of these innate responses, some infants are born with abnormally weak or intense innate responses which are likely to have a significant impact on the rearing practices of some parents. For example, an infant who does not cuddle or smile easily is likely to be ignored and neglected by the adults around him.

It has been postulated that the psychological problems of a deprived infant are the result of an unsatisfactory or nonexistent attachment to the mother. It takes a human infant about 6 to 8 months to recognize his mother, as manifested by the appearance of stranger anxiety. Fear of strangers appears at about 6 months of age in American infants, shows a peak frequency at 8 months, then gradually vanishes by the time the child is 12 to 15 months old.

Is the biologic mother necessary for the development of attachment?

It seems reasonable to hypothesize that the biologic mother is the best person with whom to develop this attachment relationship but that a surrogate mother could also develop this bond as long as she elicited the infant's primary reactions and provided food and physical comfort. Data on the rearing of adopted infants generally support this hypothesis.

It has not yet been established whether continuous care of an infant by one adult exclusively is more conducive to better social and sexual development than care by multiple parties. This is a very controversial issue. Some experts feel that excessive attachment to one set of parents may eventually result in overly individualized and aggressive behavior. Other investigators believe that mothering by several caretakers is detrimental to the development of normal social and emotional relationships.

Hospitalism

The term "hospitalism" is generally restricted to extreme cases of emotional deprivation in early infancy. Although such extreme deprivation most frequently occurs in institutions that provide long-term care to infants, this condition is also seen in home-reared infants. It is not uncommon to observe many such deprived children admitted to childrens' hospitals every year.

Infants who have experienced extreme emotional deprivation are listless and lethargic. They do not smile or babble. They often look at the passerby with wide open eyes and without any expression of feeling on their faces. They do not feel as much pain as normal infants do. Once these infants are recognized by the staff and are given a great deal of attention and care, however, they begin to change for the better. Initially, they become irritable and respond to strangers with anxiety and fear. They seem to feel more pain and cry more often. But they do manifest some attachment to the adults who spend a great deal of time with them, and if the special attention and care are continued, more pleasant emotions develop, which are expressed by smiles and babbling. Unfortunately, many of these infants are not recognized early enough by health care professionals, and their continued deprivation results in permanent damage to their emotional and intellectual faculties. Many of these children function at a retarded level as they grow older.

It should be noted that children born with a high threshold for stimulation do not benefit from normal levels of environmental stimulation and may appear to be behaviorally similar to and thus mistaken for emotionally deprived children.

Hospitalization

Tommy, an 8-year-old boy admitted to the hospital for the first time with acute abdominal pains of 2 days' duration, rings the nursing station every 5 minutes with various complaints. He is driving the nurses crazy and seems to demand everybody's attention. Are his complaints exaggerated or attention-seeking in nature?

Another boy, Jerry, 6 years old, has been admitted to the hospital for the fourth time since the onset of his first acute asthmatic attack 8 months earlier. He appears very quiet and withdrawn and does not relate much to the nurses, doctors and other children. Is he emotionally healthy?

Children admitted to hospitals react in varying ways. These psychological reactions have become a matter of genuine concern to most health care personnel, since they are likely to influence the child's response to subsequent medical care and certain aspects of the child's personality development.

As hospitals become more complex by virtue of ever-changing technology and new procedures which the layman does not understand, specific efforts must be made to simplify hospitals for parents as well as for children.

Children's hospitals formerly had limited visiting hours and were very restrictive of the parents' presence, even during minor surgical procedures. It is only since the early 1960s that visiting hours and parental involvement in the care of the hospitalized child have been liberalized. Although there are many physcians and nurses who feel uncomfortable caring for a child in the presence of parents, the parents' involvement is generally regarded as psychologically beneficial for the child as well as for the parents. There are some obvious exceptions when exclusion of the parents is warranted, however, such as when the parents are abusive, are magnifying the child's fears, or are unable to tolerate minor surgical procedures.

What is there about hospitalization that psychologically upsets children?

At least 3 factors can be recognized as contributing to a child's upset:

1. Separation from his home, parents and all his cherished belongings
2. The strangeness and unfamiliarity of the hospital
3. Fear of hospital procedures, pain, operations and mutilation

Hospitals arouse many fantasies of injury, mutilation and death in children. Some children feel they are sick because they have been bad. The sickness may thus be interpreted as punishment and abandonment.

Gellert (1961) studied 102 hospitalized and nonhospitalized children, 4 to 16 years of age. They were shown a picture of a child in bed and were asked several questions related to how the child became ill. About two thirds of the children felt that the child in the picture had been bad and had done things contrary to the expectations of his parents. These fantasies were more common among young children and children with limited intellectual capacity.

Age plays an important role in the degree of upset experienced by children, with children under 5 years old being the most upset by hospitalization because of their proneness (especially during the first 2 years of life) to stranger and separation anxieties. In addition, the young child's poor comprehension of time exaggerates the effects of a brief separation.

Every separation from the parents may create a crisis for the young infant, who may experience a severe anxiety attack when his parents leave his hospital room. This reaction is at times misinterpreted by hospital personnel, who believe it stems from the parents spoiling the child and who, accordingly, try to curtail the parents' visits to the child. These upsets usually decrease during hospitalization, however, so no curtailment of parental visiting is necessary.

The nature of the parent-child relationship also influences the child's reaction to hospitalization. Children who trust their parents are able to trust other adults, doctors and nurses. A poor and untrusting relationship between the child and his parents decreases the child's ability to trust other adults and enhances his upset when hospitalized.

The parents' own response to the child's illness is still another factor in the child's reaction to hospitalization. Many parents feel guilty about their child's illness and may overprotect him to the point of treating him as if he were an infant. A high level of parental anxiety interferes with effective psychological preparation of the child for hospitalization or surgical procedures. The lack of full comprehension of the disease or a diagnostic procedure, lack of trust in the doctor and unfamiliarity with the hospital routine are some of the contributory factors to the parents' high level of anxiety. Parental anxiety is easily communicated to the child, who, lacking understanding of the situation, may become more apprehensive than his parents.

Johnson (1955) studied the relationships between parental attitude toward illness and the behavior and attitude of children during hospitalization. He found the following: (1) a guilty attitude on the part of parents may lead the child to hate the parents, (2) an attitude of calamity on the part of parents may burden the child with groundless fears, (3) a selfish attitude on the part of parents may make the child feel rejected and (4) an oversolicitous attitude on the part of parents may lead the child to use his illness as a psychological tool with which to manipulate them.

Lelong and Lebovici (1955) reported that guilt feelings may cause some parents to ignore their child, thus making the child feel rejected and abandoned.

Preparation before Hospitalization

Children who are prepared for a surgical or medical procedure generally do well during hospitalization and suffer few psychological consequences afterward. It is the joint responsibility of the parents and the physician to prepare the child before hospitalization. If the parents lack comprehension of the procedure, they will not be able to help in this joint venture. Similarly, parental ambivalence toward the procedure or parental lack of trust in the doctor will interfere with the adequate preparation of the child. The child's personality, his intellectual capacity, his fantasies about hospitals and the nature of the procedure should be taken into account during the preparation. The amount of time required for this preparation varies. Those children who become anxious about every little thing may require earlier preparation so that they will be calmed down by the time hospitalization occurs.

Numerous books have been written for parents and children to help them prepare for hospitalization and surgical procedures. The physician should be familiar with these books and should recommend the best ones to the parents.

The psychological preparation of the family by the physician should include the following:

1. Information about the surgical or medical procedure should be imparted to the child and his parents.
2. The child and his parents should be encouraged to express their feelings and fantasies about such procedures.
3. A relationship of trust and confidence should be established with the child and his parents.

To achieve these goals, an interview is held with the parents and the child. The child is likely to ask more questions when his parents are with him. Sometimes, parents have questions that they do not feel comfortable asking in the presence of their child. They should be given an opportunity to talk with the physician privately or should be allowed to call the physician to discuss these questions.

Many hospitals have an organized program for preparing children for surgical procedures, in which the various members of the surgical team—doctors, nurses, anesthesiologist—and the patient participate in puppet or doll play. These programs are effectively carried out by trained volunteers and have been regarded as highly successful in preparing children for surgical procedures.

Day Care for Infants

Until recently, there was little research on the effects of day care on young children. By definition, day care involves separating the child from its mother for all or part of the day. For a long time, maternal separation was considered tantamount to maternal deprivation, such deprivation appearing to have toxic long-range effects if it occurred during the first 3 years of life. Thus, at the policy level, day care for the child under 3—and, by inference, employment for his mother—was discouraged. No government resources were allocated to the planning of facilities and programs for infants.

But the need for day care became more urgent. In June 1958, there were 883,000 children under 3 years of age whose mothers were employed full time. By March 1967, the number had increased to 1,024,000. Of this total, 471,000 children were cared for in their own homes, 427,000 were cared for in someone else's home, 77,000 were cared for by other arrangements, and 49,000 were in group care center programs.

Recognizing the potential importance of this problem, the U.S. Children's Bureau initiated several demonstration projects in infant care between 1964 and 1967. The projects were conducted in centers in Syracuse, New York, New Haven, Connecticut, and Greensboro, South Carolina. The young infants registered in these programs were studied for social, emotional and intellectual development.

In the Syracuse infant development project, between 1965 and 1968, 86 children who had entered day care prior to age 3 and had remained in the program for at least 6 months were compared to a control group of 34 children from a comparable social background without day care experience. Each child was tested twice, first on either the Cattell Infant Intelligence Scale or the Stanford-Binet Test, and near the end of the study period on the Stanford-Binet. Scores for the day care children increased by about 17 points, while those of control group children decreased by about 6 points.

Data from the infant center in Greensboro did not show similar cognitive gains associated with day care experience. The difference between the two studies may be explained on the basis of differences in population. Approximately two thirds of the children in the Syracuse study came from low socioeconomic groups, while the Greensboro sample consisted primarily of middle-class families.

Social and emotional development are very difficult to quantify in young children. The majority of the children involved in the various day care research projects were just reaching school age. In the Syracuse project, "attachment of children to their own mothers and the reciprocal attachment of the mothers to their children" were studied. Two different groups of mother–child dyads were observed. Children in one group of mother–child pairs had been involved in the Syracuse day care center program from the time they were approximately 1 year old. Children in the other group of 23 mother–child pairs had remained in the exclusive care of their mother during the same period. All assessments were made when the children were approximately 30 months of age. Based on observations of the interaction between the mothers and their children in a 3-hour session, interviews about the children's behavior at home and discussion of the mother's own child-rearing patterns, a cluster of ratings pertaining to attachment behavior was made for each mother and child. There were no significant differences between children in day care and home-reared children in terms of the attachment of the children to their mothers. Similarly, there were no major differences between the groups with regard to the strength of attachment of the mothers to their children.

The children were also rated on breadth of attachment, that is, their attachment to people other than their mothers. Day care infants enjoyed interacting with other people more than did home-reared children.

Because of associated health hazards like epidemics of polio or measles, it would have been foolish until just a few years ago to advocate bringing a large number of infants together in a group, but what about less serious but still troublesome illnesses?

For example, what effect does infant day care have on the incidence and severity of colds and other respiratory illnesses?

Over a 5-year period, the Greensboro research group collected data on respiratory illness among 100 preschool children who attended the center for some period of time. Most of the children entered the center before their 1st birthday. The average incidence of respiratory illness for this group was 8.9 illnesses per child per year. The highest incidence rate, 10 respiratory illnesses per year, was found among children under 1 year of age, with the incidence dropping below 8 per year among the 3 year olds.

These data were compared with data from a large metropolitan community which showed an average of 8.3 respiratory illnesses per year for

1-year-old children and 7.4 per year for children between 2 and 5 years old. They concluded that day care might be associated with a slightly higher rate of respiratory illness in children under 1 year of age but that after that age the incidence figures were very similar to those reported for home-reared children.

There are large-scale infant day care programs in Europe, the Soviet Union and Israel. Programs in Denmark suggest the following: (1) it is better to locate day care centers near the child's residence rather than the place of work of the mother, (2) small neighborhood centers are preferable to large, centralized health and social service centers, (3) children up to age 3 should be divided into 3 care groups—3–10 months, 10–18 months and 18–36 months, (4) the ratio of children to staff should vary from 2:1 to 4:1 for younger infants and increase to 8:1 for older children (5) all infant care workers should be trained, secondary school graduates who have had 1 year of specialized courses followed by a year's internship.

REFERENCES

Bakwin, H.: Loneliness in infants, Am. J. Dis. Child. 63:30, 1942.

Barry, H., Jr.: Significance of maternal bereavement before age of eight in psychiatric patients, Arch. Neurol. Psychiat. 62:630, 1949.

Bender, L., and Yarnell, H.: An observation nursery: a study of 250 children in the psychiatric division of Bellevue Hospital, Am. J. Psychiatry 97:1158, 1941.

Bowlby, J.: *Forty-four Juvenile Thieves* (London: Bailliere, Tindall and Cox, 1946).

Brown, F.: Depression and childhood bereavement, J. Ment. Sci. 107:754, 1961.

Chapin, H. D.: Are institutions for infants necessary? J.A.M.A. 64:1, 1915a.

Chapin, H. D.: A plea for accurate statistics in infants' institutions, Arch. Pediatr. 32:724, 1915b.

Durfee, H., and Wolf, K.: Anstaltspflege und Entwicklung im ersten Lebensjahr, Z. Kinderforsch. 42:273, 1933.

Gellert, E.: Children's Beliefs about Bodily Illness (Paper read at American Psychological Assoc., New York, 1961).

Glueck, S., and Glueck, E.: *Unravelling Juvenile Delinquency* (Boston: Harvard University Press, 1950).

Goldfarb, W.: Effects of early institutional care on adolescent personality, J. Exp. Educ. 12:106, 1943.

Harlow, H. F., and Harlow, M. K.: Social deprivation in monkeys, Sci. Am. 207:137, 1962.

Harlow, H. F., and Harlow, M. K.: Learning to love, Am. Sci. 54:244, 1966.

Johnson, R.: How parents' attitudes affect children's illness, Bull. Inst. Child. Stud. Toronto, 17:5, 1955.

Lelong, M., and Lebovici, S.: Psychopathologic problems posed by children in hospitals, Arch. Fr. Pediatr. 12:349, 1955.

Lorenz, K.: Der Kumpan in der Unwelt des Vogels: die Artgenosse als Auslosendes Moment, Soz. Verhaltungs Weisen J. 83:137, 1935.

Lorenz, K.: In Tanner, J. M., and Inhelder, B. (eds.): *Discussions on Child Development,* Vol. 4, (London: Tavistock, 1960), p. 128.
Lowrey, L. G.: Personality distortion and early institutional care, Am. J. Orthopsychiatry 10:576, 1940.
Spitz, R.: "Hospitalism," Psychoanal. Study Child 1:53, 1945.

2/Crisis Theory and Intervention

A CRISIS is a state of temporary disequilibrium precipitated by unavoidable life events. A person in crisis feels overwhelmed and helpless and is temporarily unable to resolve his problem by himself. In addition to anxiety, there are manifestations of cognitive uncertainty, emotional distress, psychophysiologic symptoms and disruption of social relationships.

Crises, by definition, are temporary, lasting only a few weeks. Life events that precipitate crisis may be part of normal development or external events beyond the control of the individual. These events may be obvious and easily identifiable, or they may be quite elusive. Some crisis situations are universal, such as death and fatal illness, while other situations may be experienced as crises only by certain individuals.

People differ vastly in their capacity to cope with crisis. Persons who are less vulnerable seem to possess better coping skills than individuals who are highly vulnerable. Low-vulnerable individuals are better able to reorient themselves rapidly and are able to take decisive steps in response to change and emergency situations. Highly vulnerable people, on the other hand, fall apart easily in similar situations.

Major efforts are being made, through community mental health centers and mobilization of emergency room facilities, to help people in crisis as they arrive and to resolve their problems without resorting to hospitalization. This seems especially appropriate, as the public's use of emergency rooms has increased severalfold during the last decade, and fairly large numbers of emergency room patients are not true medical emergencies. Emergency rooms and their staffs have become the primary deliverers of health care and social services. Coleman and Errera (1963) found that 5% of the patients seen in emergency room settings were clearly distinguishable as needing psychiatric consultation or treatment. In addition, there are crises associated with acute or chronic medical conditions that may go unnoticed but that may impair the normal functioning of the family.

Phases of Crisis

Studies of individuals, families and groups in crisis reveal that crisis is a regular process and that people in crisis undergo a fairly predictable sequence of emotional events. Different authors have classified these emotional events differently. Most authors, however, differentiate among and assign some significance to the beginning, middle and final stages of a crisis.

Bowlby (1952) studied infants who were separated from their mothers and were hospitalized in institutions for long periods of time. This separation was considered a crisis for the infants, who went through 3 distinct phases during the crisis—protest, despair and detachment.

Lindemann (1944) studied bereavement reactions among the survivors of those killed in the Coconut Grove night club fire and developed the fundamentals of *crisis theory* as a conceptual framework for preventive psychiatry. He noted that the duration of grief reaction depended on the success with which a person did his grief work. According to Lindemann, a normal course of grief reaction begins when the bereaved (1) begins to emancipate himself from bondage to the deceased, (2) makes a readjustment in the environment in which the deceased is missing and (3) forms new relationships or patterns of interaction that bring reward and satisfaction.

Caplan (1964) described the following 4 phases which he considered characteristic of most crisis situations:

1. There is an initial rise in tension which calls forth habitual problem-solving responses to achieve equilibrium.

2. If these problem-solving responses are not successful and the crisis continues, there is a further rise of tension and upset.

3. The individual mobilizes his reserves of strength and his emergency problem-solving mechanisms. He tries new problem-solving methods. He may gradually define the problem in a new way so that it becomes similar to previous experiences. He may compromise and give up certain aspects of the goal as unattainable. He may continue to struggle in trial-and-error fashion until all avenues are explored and the problem is resolved.

4. If the problem remains unresolved, tension mounts to dangerous levels. Manifestations of severe emotional disturbance and personality disorganization may then appear.

In studying families in crisis as a result of the birth of a premature infant, Kaplan and Mason (1960) identified the following 4 phases which he felt families needed to work through in order to resolve the crisis in a healthy manner.

1. Once the possibility of a premature birth is determined, the mother must prepare herself psychologically for a possible loss through the process of anticipatory grief.

2. Feelings of failure and inability to deliver a full-term baby should be acknowledged by the mother.

These two anticipatory processes are likely to create an emotional distance between the surviving baby and the mother.

3. Thus, if the baby survives, there must be a resumption of processes of relating to the baby.

4. Mother and father must recognize the special needs of the premature infant.

Tyhurst (1957), referring to more major disasters, identified 3 phases of a crisis—a period of impact, a period of recoil and a posttraumatic period. Elaborating on Tyhurst's formulation, Hirschowitz (1973) conceptualized a crisis sequence as involving impact, recoil–turmoil, adjustment and reconstruction.

Impact is a state of shock resulting from distressing news. The more unexpected the news, the greater the intensity of shock. The shock may last from a few hours to a few days, depending upon the subjective meaning of the experience and the availability of external support. Emotions during this phase are very intense, and the person is frequently caught between opposing drives of fight and flight. As a result of the intensity of emotion, cognitive functions and social relationships are disturbed. The individual may become easily distracted and disoriented. Severe crises may mimic acute brain syndrome.

Recoil–turmoil follows as the person assimilates the news. The dazed state during the impact phase is replaced by rage, anxiety, depression, guilt and shame, which may be expressed openly by weeping, anger and destructive behavior or may be concealed behind a facade of coolness and detachment. This phase may last from 1 to 4 weeks. Most persons become preoccupied with the past. They mourn for and reminisce about the lost person or situation.

Adjustment refers to the acceptance of the situation both cognitively and emotionally. The painful feelings become muted and are gradually tempered with hope about the future. The person begins to feel within himself: "All is not lost" and "life must go on." This phase may last for several weeks.

Reconstruction may take weeks or months. The person explores new relationships and tries new solutions to the problems that confront him. Time orientation shifts from preoccupation with the past to future possibilities and brings with it planning, new goals and a new attitude toward the future.

Factors Influencing Outcome of a Crisis

Every crisis is a new situation with its own unique set of circumstances, some of which may be familiar to the individual, while others are completely novel and require new types of coping skills. Some people resolve their crisis without any setbacks or regressions, while others emerge with a lower level of adjustment. There are still others who use crisis situations for growth and who emerge with better coping skills and a higher level of adjustment.

The outcome of a crisis depends upon many factors, such as personal strengths, familial support, sociocultural traditions and community facilities available to the person in crisis. Personal factors include the coping skills of the individual and his past experience with similar problems. If the present crisis is symbolically linked to or explicitly similar to a past crisis, it is important to determine how well the person dealt with and solved the previous crisis. If the person successfully dealt with the previous crisis, he is likely to succeed again. Past experience with similar problems reduces the probability of a problem becoming a new crisis. On the other hand, unsuccessfully resolved past crises are likely to result in repetition of previously unsuccessful solutions before new solutions are found.

A person does not face crisis alone. He is helped or hindered by the people around him, his family, his friends and his cultural traditions. Different cultures vary in the degree of tolerance they show to people in crisis. Similarly, different family members provide varying amounts of support. Immediate availability of social and psychological services to people in crisis helps assure a favorable outcome.

Events Causing Crisis

It is difficult to predict with certainty which life events will produce crisis in which individuals, for not all individuals faced with the same crisis event will enter a state of crisis. On the other hand, there are certain universal events, such as death, that will create crisis in most individuals, though of different intensity and duration. Physical illness and monetary problems are likely to intensify reactions to a crisis. Groups or families facing a crisis together generally fare much better than individuals facing the crisis alone.

Holmes (1978) studied a large number of life events and assigned a value to each life event on the basis of its stressful impact on the individual (Table 2–1).

Healthy and Unhealthy Crisis Coping

Individuals in crisis utilize a habitual mode of problem-solving which they have used successfully in the past. Crises are often novel situations, however, and may not be amenable to old problem-solving methods but may require new problem-solving techniques.

TABLE 2-1.—RATING LIFE CHANGE

LIFE EVENT	VALUE
Death of spouse	100
Divorce	73
Marital separation	65
Jail term	63
Death of close family member	63
Personal injury or illness	53
Marriage	50
Fired at work	47
Marital reconciliation	45
Retirement	45
Change in health of family member	44
Pregnancy	40
Sex difficulties	39
Gain of new family member	39
Change in financial state	38
Death of a close friend	37
Change to different line of work	36
Change in number of arguments with spouse	35
Mortgage over $10,000	31
Foreclosure of mortgage or loan	30

Based on data from Holmes, T. H.: Psychosomatics 19: 747, 1978.

Hirschowitz (1973) identifies the following behaviors as characteristic of people who cope well with crisis:

1. Such a person is able to deal simultaneously with both the affective dimensions of his experience and the tasks that confront him. He is aware of his painful emotions and gives them appropriate expression but does not engage in interminable catharsis or ventilation. As he expresses his pain, he frees energy for mastery of his environmental challenges. Crisis mastery proceeds by the conversion of uncertainty into manageable risk. This process of situational mastery is crucial. When life change is anticipated, this intelligent worry work can begin in advance, with significant diminution of the intensity of the crisis. Programs of anticipatory guidance or emotional prophylaxis incorporate these principles of anticipatory planning and action rehearsal.

2. He has the ability to acknowledge his increased dependency needs and to seek, receive and use assistance.

3. He values the active mastery of environmental challenges and recognizes their value in promoting increased understanding and personal growth.

4. In coping with anxieties, he uses such defenses as substitution and modes of tension relief that do not have destructive consequences.

The person who copes badly with crisis has some or all of the following traits:

1. He exhibits excessive denial, withdrawal, retreat or avoidance, with fantasy replacing or merging with reality.
2. His behavior is often impulsive, and he ventilates his rage on vulnerable, relatively powerless family members who lend themselves to being scapegoats.
3. He meets his dependency needs by excessive clinging or counterdependent avoidance of assistance. These patterns, described by Bowlby as protest, despair and detachment, resemble the behavior of separated infants. These actions are either annoying or indicate to others that the individual neither wants nor needs help; thus they do not usually evoke ministration responses from others.
4. He denies and overcontrols his emotions, with eventual eruption of suppressed feelings.
5. His malcoping may assume the form of the hopelessness-helplessness-giving-up syndrome described by Engel (1954) and his associates.
6. He may resort to hyperritualistic behavior, which serves little or no purpose.
7. His rest-work cycle is poorly regulated, due to the fatigue of the crisis state.
8. He may rely on magic by mouth, with recourse to pain-reducing substances, such as drugs or alcohol, or adopt an addictive pattern of compulsive food intake.
9. He cannot ask for help and cannot use it when it is offered.

Crisis As Opportunity

Concepts such as "stress" or "trauma" frequently carry a negative connotation. Stress is generally considered a burden or a load under which a person may crack up. Stress has been assumed to have a pathogenic potential and to give rise to all kinds of emotional problems.

This theory of stress does not account for the common phenomenon that individuals who succeed in mastering a distressing experience often appear stronger and are better able to deal effectively in the future not only with the same stress but with other difficulties as well. Some soldiers, for example, break down under the stress of combat and develop combat neurosis, while other soldiers are strengthened by combat experience and emerge with increased self-reliance and improved capacity for leadership and initiative.

Stimulation of personal growth by exposure to small doses of stress and challenge has long been successfully used by educators and scout leaders.

Although crisis is often used interchangeably with stress, it is usually equated with great amounts of stress and disaster. Crisis creates a serious problem for the individual in his current life situation. The problem may be experienced or conceived of as a threat, a loss or a challenge. If the problem is viewed as a challenge, it is more likely to be met with a mobilization of energy and purposeful problem-solving activities.

Thomas (Volkhart, 1951) perceives crisis as a catalyst that disrupts old habits, evokes new responses and becomes a major factor in the creation of new actions. Crises elicit new coping mechanisms, thus strengthening the individual's adaptive capacity and, thereby, generally raising his level of mental health.

Tyhurst (1957) equates crisis with an opportunity for growth. A crisis requires a solution which is new in relation to the individual's previous life experience. Many individuals are able to develop new solutions by means of the normal range of problem-solving mechanisms and are, thereby, able to deal adequately with the crisis. Others are unable to develop appropriate solutions, and, for them, the crisis continues to be a source of stress.

Crisis is viewed by most authors as a transitional period, presenting an individual either with the opportunity for personal growth or with the danger of increased vulnerability to mental disorders. Crisis often gives a person a second chance to correct overly relied-upon but faulty problem-solving techniques or to develop new problem-solving strategies more appropriate to the new situation. Resistance to mental disorder can be strengthened by helping individuals extend their repertoire of effective problem-solving skills so that they will not need to use regressive, non-reality-based or socially unacceptable ways of dealing with stressful situations, which often lead to the development of neurotic or psychotic symptoms.

Types of Crisis

Crisis may be divided into 2 broad categories: developmental and situational. Personality development is generally described as a succession of differentiated phases, each qualitatively different from its predecessor. Between one phase and the next are transitional periods which are characterized by cognitive and emotional turbulence. These periods have been called "developmental crises" (Erikson, 1959). Developmental (or maturational) crises thus occur during various stages of normal development.

Situational crises, on the other hand, are precipitated primarily by stressful events that occur in a person's life situation and threaten his integrity and equilibrium. Some of the events that precipitate situational crisis, such as rape, physical illness, suicidal attempts and death, are discussed elsewhere in this book. Other events that have been studied extensively include the possibility or actual birth of a premature baby, divorce and separation, and running away from home.

Although the number of maturational crises in an individual's life may be innumerable, certain crisis situations have been better defined and more clearly recognized than others during the various stages of development. For example, in infancy, separation of the baby from the mother creates a crisis for the baby. The infant goes through the phases of protest, despair and withdrawal. If the separation is continued without the development of other attachments, the infant may become severely withdrawn and suffer anaclitic depression. Other minor crises occur when the baby develops stranger anxiety and separation anxiety. Stranger anxiety normally occurs in American children between 6 and 8 months of age and lasts until about 12 months of age. Separation anxiety makes its appearance between 10 and 12 months of age in American children and begins to disappear by the time the child is 20 to 24 months old.

Some parents who are ignorant of the normal maturational problems of children during the early stages of development push their children to socialize with strangers and separate themselves forcibly from the child without giving much support to the child and without regard to the traumatic effects of their actions. It is not uncommon for these children to be whiny and clinging and still subject to stranger and separation anxieties.

Entering nursery school or kindergarten presents another crisis situation for the young child. School phobia is not an uncommon occurrence in children who have not been prepared well for this separation from the parents and for socialization with their peers.

Pronounced fear of death has sometimes been referred to as "8-year anxiety" because it tends to be fairly common at this age. In a considerable number of children, there occurs at this age what Anthony (1967) calls "existential crisis." The child becomes increasingly preoccupied with ideas that either he or his parents will die. The child's concept of death, like many of his other ideas, develops gradually during the early years. Before the age of 7, death is seen as reversible. At about 8 years of age for many children, death is perceived as irreversible. The child becomes aware of a particular kind of helplessness in the face of the inevitability of death. Actual experience of the death of a significant other may sometimes be instrumental in precipitating a death phobia.

The onset of puberty and adolescence presents another developmental crisis. There is a revival and reassessment of earlier emotional ties with parents and other significant adults. There are many small emotional crises during this stage of development. The adolescent strives to become independent and to acquire his own identity. Some adolescents, however, seem to continue this quest for identity throughout their adolescence. They seem to be confused and to have a great deal of difficulty in acquiring clear-cut roles for themselves.

Crisis Intervention

Crisis intervention is a therapeutic technique designed to help the person in crisis. Its goal is to fully or partially resolve the crisis and to restore the individual or family to the level of functioning that existed before the crisis. Recent developments in ego psychology have contributed a great deal to the evolution of this type of therapy. Crisis intervention techniques focus on coping with present ego disintegration rather than on acquiring insight into unconscious conflicts.

A crisis is a state in which there is a disintegration of personality and a breakdown of habitual modes of coping. During a crisis, a person is less defensive and more open to outside influences because he is more dependent upon others for understanding, emotional support and guidance in solving or seeking new solutions to real, identifiable problems.

Since the crisis is characteristically self-limiting, lasting 4 to 6 weeks, time is at a premium, and an immediate therapeutic climate should be created. The intervenor must possess knowledge of and competency in problem-solving techniques and must be capable of guiding and supporting his client. This does not mean that the therapist will have the answer to every problem. He is expected, however, to understand the sequence of events in crisis resolution and to plan a series of therapeutic steps to bring about the resolution.

Several therapeutic approaches have been outlined by different authors. Jacobson and associates (1968) suggest 2 main approaches to crisis intervention: generic and individual.

The generic approach focuses upon the characteristic course of a particular kind of crisis rather than on the psychodynamics of each individual in that crisis. Specific intervention measures are designed to be effective for all members of a given group rather than being tailor-made for each specific individual. This approach is based on the assumption that there are certain patterns of behavior which are common in most crises. Many studies have substantiated this thesis. Lindemann's work on bereavement (1944) indicates, for example, that there is a well-defined process that a person goes through in adjusting to the death of a relative. This process, called "grief work," includes preoccupation with the image of the deceased person and then a gradual detachment from the deceased person and an emotional attachment to new persons.

The generic approach emphasizes: (1) specific situational and maturational events occurring to significant population groups and (2) intervention oriented to crises resulting from these specific events. The generic approach to crisis intervention consists of specific measures designed to be effective for the group as a whole, such as direct encouragement of adaptive behavior, general support, environmental manipulation and anticipatory guidance.

The individual approach to crisis intervention differs from the generic approach by virtue of its emphasis on professional assessment of the specific intrapsychic and interpersonal habits of the individual in crisis. This approach also differs from traditional psychotherapy by virtue of its lack of concern with a thorough understanding of psychodynamic processes except as they provide clues that aid in understanding the current crisis. It focuses solely on why and how a previous equilibrium has been disturbed and on the processes involved in reaching a new equilibrium. A second difference from conventional therapy is the inclusion of other family members in the crisis intervention. The individual approach is not the therapy of choice when the crisis affects a family or a group of people. It is used in selected cases, especially when the individual in crisis presents an unusual pattern of response to the crisis or has not responded to the generic approach. The individual approach emphasizes the need for deeper and more detailed understanding of the individual's coping pattern and the necessity of tailoring intervention to the individual's unique situation.

Another approach to crisis intervention, suggested by Hansell et al. (1970) and called "decision counseling," involves the following steps:

1. Identify all the events causing the crisis.
2. Make an innovative list of all possible options and alternatives.
3. Help the patient select a definite alternative from among the options.
4. Encourage the patient to try out his option in real life.
5. Assess the outcome of the trial, and start over with another option if the first one was not satisfactory.

The authors of decision counseling emphasize that the mood and emotional life of people undergo dramatic improvement as decisions are made, especially decisions which have been pending a long time or about which the individual has been frightened or pessimistic. Introducing more options for consideration maximizes the opportunity for flexibility, enhances individuality and minimizes the likelihood of a short-term crisis becoming a long-term status quo.

Steps in Crisis Intervention

Crisis intervention should not be considered a second best therapy but rather the treatment of choice with persons in crisis. An accurate assessment of the presenting problem is essential to effective crisis intervention. It is a time-limited approach, during which therapeutic efforts are directed toward resolution of the presenting problems. It is important to remember that dealing with matters that are not directly related to the crisis has no place in this kind of intervention. The intervenor should play an active role in directing and guiding his patients. Morley and associates (1967) have outlined the following steps:

1. The first phase of crisis intervention involves the assessment of the individual and his problem. Persons with severe suicidal or homocidal potentials are referred for individual evaluation and possible hospitalization.

Of critical importance in crisis intervention is the accurate assessment of the precipitating event and the resulting crisis that brought the individual to treatment. Often the first hour is devoted entirely to this assessment.

2. Next, the nature of the therapeutic intervention is planned. This planning depends upon several factors, such as the amount of time elapsed since the onset of the crisis, the coping skills of the individual, the degree of support offered by the family, the ego strength of the individual prior to onset of the crisis and the degree to which the person's life has been disrupted.

3. The third step is the intervention itself. The therapist may utilize any number of techniques with which he is familiar, as long as he keeps in mind the basic philosophy and goal of crisis intervention. Morley has found the following techniques useful:

(a) Help the individual to gain an intellectual understanding of his crisis. Many individuals may have no idea that there is a relationship between some life event and their feelings of extreme discomfort and crisis. The therapist should actively help the patient understand the relationship between the precipitating events and his state of crisis.

(b) Help the person to talk about his present situation and his associated feelings. It is not uncommon for people in crisis to suppress such socially unacceptable feelings as anger, hate, aggression and guilt. The therapist should be uncritical, accepting and encouraging of such feelings.

(c) Explore the coping behaviors and techniques that the person is using to deal with the present crisis. Also explore the coping behaviors and techniques that the person utilized in the past in similar situations. The therapist should point out the ineffectiveness of the present coping behaviors and techniques and may suggest alternate ones.

(d) Reopen the social world. When there has been loss of a significant

person in an individual's life, the introduction of new people or old friends into the patient's social life may be highly effective.

4. The final step is the resolution of the crisis and anticipatory planning. As anxiety and depression subside and the person begins to readjust his daily life, the therapist should reinforce the change and help the individual experience the gains he has made. Help is also given in making realistic plans for the future.

Therapeutic Methods

Group therapy and family therapy have been heavily utilized by therapists doing crisis intervention therapy. These modalities of treatment, however, have been greatly modified to meet the objectives of crisis intervention. Crisis groups and crisis family therapy are common modalities of treatment utilized in crisis intervention clinics.

CRISIS GROUPS.—These groups may include members of the patient's family and friends or may consist of strangers unrelated to the patient. Crisis groups may be designed on the basis of the generic approach to crisis intervention. In this approach, the group members are chosen on the basis of having experienced a similar type of crisis, such as divorce, separation, death or drug addiction. Such groups may be open-ended or closed. The closed groups are run for a limited period of time, such as 6 to 8 weeks, with the same members attending all the sessions. In open-ended groups, new members are added as they arrive, but the number of group sessions that a member can attend is limited.

Crisis groups may be formed using individuals who are experiencing acute problems of a varied and heterogeneous nature. Such groups are formed in the belief that the group members will benefit from interacting with each other and will learn from one another's experience of coping with acute crises.

Whatever the composition of the group, the goal of the crisis group remains the same—that is, helping each individual to resolve his crisis and to restore his equilibrium. The members of the group and the therapist explore the precipitating events and present coping skills and alternate ways of dealing with the crisis. The group remains focused on the here and now, and detailed discussions of past history are discouraged.

The therapist functions as a participating leader. He actively participates in the discussions and provides direction and guidance to various members of the group. Passive and nonparticipating members should be actively encouraged to talk about their experience.

Many individuals who refuse traditional therapy will not object to participating in a short-term therapy group. Many therapists, however, feel that the time limitation is a disadvantage, as a 6 to 8 week period does not allow for the analysis of group processes, and the discussion of problems by group members remains at a superficial level. The open-endedness of a group often creates loss of continuity and greater need for repetition, since members are constantly changing, and new members must be brought up to date on the problem areas of others.

CRISIS FAMILY THERAPY.—When a particular family member becomes a psychiatric patient, other members of the family invariably become involved in his problems. They may contribute to the intensity of the patient's problems, or the patient's illness may create an emotional crisis for them. Although crisis family therapy is frequently used to keep the patient out of the hospital during an acute crisis, the seriousness of the problem may be such that the family is not able to deal with the patient, and the patient has to be hospitalized. Even in these circumstances, family therapy is likely to reduce the patient's stay in the hospital.

Crisis family therapy is also used to help families with common crises, such as the death of a member of the family, family discord and severe physical illness. At times, family therapy can be provided in anticipation of a crisis, such as birth of a premature infant or movement of the family from one part of the country to another.

Pittman and associates (1966) have outlined a technique for crisis family therapy under the following headings:

1. Immediate aid. Crisis family therapy is provided as soon as a family is recognized to be in crisis. Family treatment unit team members are always on call. They should be available around the clock, 7 days a week.

2. Defining the crisis as a family problem. The family is seen together for the first session. They are told that the existing crisis is a family problem and that all members of the family must work together to resolve the crisis. Extended members of the family as well as representatives of other agencies involved with the family are invited to work with the family treatment unit team.

3. Focus on current crisis. The problems of the current crisis are kept at the center of attention. The factors precipitating the crisis are intensively searched for and scrutinized. Members of the family are helped to acquire a cognitive understanding of the relationship between the precipitating events and the resulting crisis.

4. General prescription. Although specific approaches to family therapy have been described in special crisis situations, such as bereavement (Lindemann, 1944) and birth of a premature child (Rapaport, 1963), most family crises are dealt with via a general approach of helping the family understand the causes of the crisis, reducing their tension and gradually

resolving the crisis. High tension and severe depression in family members should be treated with appropriate medication.

5. Specific prescription. It is assumed that a series of events within the family has deleteriously affected a vulnerable and susceptible member of the family. These events begin with a change in family equilibrium. This change in equilibrium may be due to a change in family composition (e.g., birth of a new baby or visit of an in-law), a change in the role of a family member (e.g., wife going back to work after many years of full-time housekeeping) or a change in the circumstances of the family requiring a new role (e.g., serious illness of one member forcing other members to earn a living). Such changes require a reshuffling of the roles of almost all members of the family to varying degrees. Crisis occurs when there is resistance to the adoption of new roles or when an important role is left unfilled.

On the basis of his understanding of the precipitating events, the therapist may assign specific tasks to different members of the family on a trial basis.

6. Identification of role conflicts and renegotiation. It is not uncommon to find family members who are involved in role conflict with the patient. These role conflicts should be identified and discussed in the family sessions. Conflicting roles are negotiated and clarified for the conflicting parties.

7. Termination. The number of family sessions combined with some home visits may range from 6 to 8 sessions for most crisis situations. The intervention is designed to restore the equilibrium of the family to its pre-crisis level. Many long-term problems which become apparent during crisis family therapy are not resolved and may require referral for further treatment. For example, an ongoing marital problem may require referral to a marriage counselor.

Termination is carried out on an open-door policy, that is, the family may come back as they feel the need for treatment. Follow-up through telephone contact and clinic visits scheduled every few months for a period of one year have been found helpful in keeping these families out of crisis.

REFERENCES

Anthony, E. J.: Psychoneurotic Disorders, in Freedman, A. M., and Kaplan, H. I. (eds.): *Comprehensive Textbook of Psychiatry* (Baltimore: Williams and Wilkins, 1967).

Bowlby, J.: *Maternal Care and Mental Health.* (Geneva: World Health Organization, 1952).

Caplan, G.: *Principles of Preventive Psychiatry* (New York: Basic Books, Inc., 1964).

Coleman, J. V., and Errera, P.: The general hospital emergency room and its psychiatric problems, Am. J. Public Health 53:1294, 1963.

Engel, G. L.: Studies of ulcerative colitis. I. Clinical data bearing on the nature of the somatic process, Psychosom. Med. 16:496, 1954.

Erikson, E. H.: *Growth and Crises of the Healthy Personality in Identity and the Life Cycle,* Psychological Issues, Vol. 1, no. 1, Monograph 1 (New York: International University Press, 1959).

Hansell, N., Wodarczyk, M., and Lathrop, B. H.: Decision counseling method, Arch. Gen. Psychiatry 22:462, 1970.

Hirschowitz, R. G.: Crisis theory: a formulation, Psychiatry Ann. 3:33, 1973.

Holmes, T. H.: Life situations, emotions, and disease, Psychosomatics 19:747, 1978.

Jacobson, G. F., Strickler, M., and Morley, W. E.: Generic and individual approaches to crisis intervention, Am. J. Public Health 58:338, 1968.

Kaplan, D. M., and Mason, E. A.: Maternal reactions to premature birth viewed as an acute emotional disorder, Am. J. Orthopsychiatry 30:539, 1960.

Lindemann, E.: Symptomatology and management of acute grief, Am. J. Psychiatry 101:141, 1944.

Morley, W. E., Messick, J. M., and Aguilera, D. C.: Crisis: Paradigms of intervention, J. Psychiatr. Nurs. 5:531, 1967.

Pittman, F., Flomenhaft, K., DeYoung, C., Kaplan, J., and Langsley, D.: Techniques of Family Crisis Therapy, in Masserman, J. (ed.): *Current Psychiatric Therapies* (New York: Grune & Stratton, 1966).

Rapaport, R.: Normal crisis, family structure, and mental health, Fam. Process 2:68, 1963.

Tyhurst, J.: The Role of Transition States Including Disasters in Mental Illness, Symposium on Preventive and Social Psychiatry, Walter Reed Army Institute of Research, Washington, D.C., 1957.

Volkhart, E. (ed.): *Social Behavior and Personality Contributions of W. I. Thomas to Theory and Social Research* (New York: Social Science Research Council, 1951).

3/Acute Symptoms—Organic or Psychological?

ACUTE SYMPTOMS of pain, vomiting, anorexia, diarrhea, fainting, palpitation, hyperventilation and bronchospasm can result from either organic or psychological causes. The management of acute symptoms is undertaken first on the assumption of an organic etiology. A psychological diagnosis is made only after the search for organic causes is exhausted and has proved negative. There are a few syndromes, such as anorexia nervosa, tension headache and hyperventilation syndrome, however, in which a psychological etiology is usually postulated, as no organic etiology has yet been detected. Investigation and acceptance of psychological factors vary a great deal among physicians. In many teaching hospitals the diagnostic work-up of certain diseases routinely includes psychological investigation, while in other hospitals psychiatric consultation is sought only after organic etiology has been ruled out.

What can psychiatry contribute to the diagnostic work-up of a postulated psychosomatic illness?

How does a psychiatrist arrive at a diagnosis of psychogenic etiology?

Amost all illnesses have, at one time or another, been regarded as psychogenic in origin. The following classification of psychophysiologic disorders includes disorders that may occur in different physiologic systems:

1. Psychophysiologic skin disorders—include neurodermatosis, pruritis, atopic dermatitis and hyperhydrosis
2. Psychophysiologic musculoskeletal disorders—include backache, muscle cramps, myalgias and tension headaches
3. Psychophysiologic respiratory disorders—include bronchial asthma, hyperventilation syndrome, sighing and hiccups
4. Psychophysiologic cardiovascular disorders—include paroxysmal tachycardia, hypertension, vascular spasm and migraine
5. Psychophysiologic gastrointestinal disorders—include peptic ulcer, chronic gastritis, ulcerative colitis, constipation, hyperacidity, pylorospasm, heartburn and irritable colon
6. Psychophysiologic genitourinary disorders—include disturbances of menstruation and micturition, dyspareunia and impotence

7. Psychophysiologic disorders of the senses—include psychological disturbances of eyesight, hearing, smell or taste

Few physicians believe that the diseases listed above are caused entirely by psychogenic factors. This skepticism is fully justified because of the absence of compelling scientific data confirming the relationship between psychological factors and the onset of these diseases. The discussion of these diseases is further complicated by the imprecise use of terminology. The term "psychosomatic" is frequently used to refer to all the psychological factors that influence the body. These psychological factors may actually produce the illness or may simply accompany or be a response to the disease. A distinction is frequently made between psychophysiologic disorders and conversion reactions. Conversion reactions are disorders that occur in the sensory motor system of the body and are exemplified by paralysis, loss of sensation, blindness and hearing difficulties. Psychophysiologic disorders occur in the organs innervated by the autonomic nervous system.

The exact mechanisms of psychophysiologic disorders and conversion reactions are not known. Several theories have been advanced to explain the mechanism by which emotions influence bodily organs. Alexander (1950) stated that psychosomatic symptoms result from physiologic concomitants of psychic conflict in the following manner:

Psychic event → emotional arousal → associated physiologic events → dysfunction of physiologic functions → symptoms

However, not every person experiencing grief, rage or anxiety will develop psychosomatic symptoms. The manifestation of such symptoms depends upon individual susceptibility. Some individuals are highly vulnerable and will develop symptoms in response to almost any sort of emotional arousal, while others will develop symptoms only when emotional arousal becomes excessive.

Theories that combine psyche and soma emphasize that psychological and physiologic variables represent different aspects of affect and that there is a continuous feedback between central and peripheral mechanisms. Individual susceptibility to psychophysiologic disorders may be influenced by such multiple factors as constitution, nutritional status and organ pathology.

Why do different people react to a similar psychological event or emotion with different symptoms, such as peptic ulcer, ulcerative colitis, bronchospasm or hypertension?

Three psychological models have been advanced to explain this phenomenon: (1) specificity model, (2) nonspecificity model and (3) individual response specificity model.

Specificity Model

The specificity model states that specific psychic events lead to specific affective states, which are associated with specific psychophysiologic symptoms. There are several proponents of this model. Dunbar (1954) attempted to correlate specific personality profiles with specific psychophysiologic disorders. For example, it is commonly believed that a hard-driving personality type is more vulnerable to coronary artery disease. Such correlations, however, have not received incontrovertible scientific corroboration. Wolf and Wolff (1943) investigated the relationship between various physiologic and psychological parameters in healthy subjects as well as in patients suffering from various psychophysiologic illnesses. They found that certain specific attitudes held by the patient were more common in certain diseases, e.g., an attitude of grimly holding on was unusually prevalent in individuals with psychogenic constipation and diarrhea.

Alexander (1950) applied psychoanalytic theory to understanding psychophysiologic disorders. He emphasized that the arousal of specific unconscious conflict gives rise to specific psychophysiologic symptoms in the following sequence:

> Psychologic event → unconscious conflict (felt as anxiety) → regression to earlier stages of development (to the stage at which the conflict originated or the person was fixated) → specific physiologically immature reactions (pathologic pattern of arousal)

According to this model, for example, peptic ulcer patients invariably suffer from unresolved unconsicous conflict over dependency needs which have their roots in the oral period. When this neurotic conflict is reactivated by external frustrations, the patient regresses to the oral receptive stage, which is characterized by an unconscious wish to be fed by the mother. The physiologic response accompanying this psychological regression takes the form of gastric hypersecretion. If such a psychophysiologic constellation is chronically activated in an orally fixated person with vulnerable duodenal mucosa, peptic ulcer may result. According to this hypothesis, peptic ulcers do not develop in the absence of this specific unconscious conflict.

Nonspecificity Model

According to this model, psychosomatic disorders can be precipitated by any event that arouses an emotional reaction. Mahl's theory (1953,

1954) states that any stressful event may evoke a state of chronic anxiety whose physiologic concomitants will be identical, irrespective of the nature of the precipitating event. It postulates that the nature of the psychophysiologic symptoms cannot be predicted on the basis of specific psychological considerations and states that sufficient data are not yet available to explain why a particular organ becomes dysfunctional. Such organ selection may depend upon factors as yet inadequately understood or conceptualized, such as constitutional organ susceptibility and early psychological experiences.

Individual Response Specificity Model

Many individuals show highly characteristic and consistent physiologic patterns of emotional arousal to a wide range of events or stimuli, with the same stimulus triggering increased heart rate or palpitation in one person but increased gastric secretion in another. Thus, according to their predominant response, people can be labeled "cardiac reactors," "gastric reactors" or "hypertensive reactors." An individual's characteristic response pattern is established in early childhood and is highly consistent over time. Malmo (1962) has presented evidence that different physiologic patterns of emotional arousal are associated with specific psychosomatic symptoms and diseases.

Diagnosis of Psychophysiologic Disorders

Few psychophysiologic syndromes are universally accepted as having an entirely psychogenic etiology. There are, however, many illnesses which are believed to have a psychological component in their etiology. The diagnosis of most of the so-called psychophysiologic illnesses, such as peptic ulcer, ulcerative colitis and essential hypertension, is made primarily by internists or other medical specialists. The psychiatrist is usually consulted only to provide psychological treatment, though at times he may be called upon to help diagnose certain borderline conditions, such as recurrent abdominal pain, fainting spells, headache and anorexia nervosa.

Depending upon his theoretical bias, the psychiatrist tries to determine the identity, intensity and sources of the stresses that may have precipitated the illness. He does this by obtaining a clinical history from the parents, including the child's personal, social and familial adjustment, and by interviewing the child. Care must be taken to distinguish between the emotional stress that precipitated the illness and the stress that occurs as a response to the illness. It is generally assumed that any person with severe social and familial problems is especially vulnerable to psychophysiologic illness. This assumption, however, is unwarranted, since major differences exist in the coping capacities and capabilities of individuals.

Specific psychodynamics have been reported for each of the psychophysiologic illnesses. The formulation of such dynamics from the initial interview is frequently very difficult, and several sessions with the child and family are usually required before the specific psychodynamics of the disease become apparent.

Each physiologic system is unique in its response to psychological stress. The intensity and the nature of the pathology caused by stress vary from one system to another.

How does psychological stress cause pathology in various organs?

Although much research has been devoted to the psychophysiologic relationship between psychological stress and organ pathology, the level and accuracy of understanding achieved to date remain primitive. The following sections summarize our current knowledge in this area.

Gastrointestinal Tract

PSYCHOPHYSIOLOGY.—The gastrointestinal tract (GIT) is richly innervated by the sympathetic and the parasympathetic nervous systems. The normal physiologic functions of the GIT, such as variations in the tone of smooth muscle and changes in motility and secretion, have been shown to be influenced by various emotional states. Emotions are presumed to influence gastrointestinal functions by activating the higher autonomic centers in the brain.

The most common psychophysiologic disorders involving the esophagus are globus hystericus and cardiospasm. In globus hystericus, there is a sensation of fullness in the throat and difficulty in the initiation of swallowing. Studies of the patient with globus hystericus show that there are no changes in the motility of the esophagus, and the pharynx is usually clear and empty. Faulkner (1940), through studies with barium swallow, demonstrated that narrowing or complete obliteration of the esophageal lumen may occur in response to different types of suggested emotions, such as grief, anger and anxiety.

Although some cases of cardiospasm are accompanied by structural changes with absence of myenteric ganglia in the lower esophagus, temporary conditions of cardiospasm are much more frequent than can be accounted for by permanent structural changes. Some cases of cardiospasm seem to follow an acute emotional upset. Wolf and Almy (1949) noted an increased esophageal transport time in response to noxious stimuli. Rubin et al. (1962) demonstrated that, in normal subjects, intraesophageal pressure changes were related to the emotional state of the individual.

Several studies have investigated the relationship among various emotional states and gastric secretion, motor activity and vascular supply. The classic studies of Wolf and Wolff (1943) on their patient, Tom, elucidated many of these relationships. Tom was an ideal subject because he had a gastric fistula, and, therefore, the investigators were able to collect gastric secretion and to observe the vascularity and fragility of the gastric mucosa. The influence of emotional states on Tom's gastric functions was studied for several years. The authors noted that in states of hostility and resentment, there was usually increased gastric secretion, as measured by hydrochloric acid production; increased mucosal blood flow, as measured by mucosal color; and increased gastric motility, as measured by an intragastric balloon or gastric emptying time. The mucosal fragility of gastric stoma was increased during periods of gastric hyperfunction, as evidenced by the small ulcers which could be produced on the exposed gastric mucosa by minimal trauma. States of depression and dejection produced diminished gastric secretion, decreased vascular supply and decreased motility. It was noted also that, during periods of depressed gastric functions, the expected response of the stomach to a physiologic or pharmacologic stimulus was diminished. For example, the usual response of the stomach to the ingestion of beef broth (increased secretion) was diminished in depression.

Kehoe and Ironside (1963) induced various emotional states by means of hypnosis. They too found that the gastric secretion was increased in states of anger and anxiety and decreased in depression and states of helplessness and hopelessness.

Margolin et al. (1950) studied a patient, named Helen, who had a gastric fistula. They noted that gastric secretion either increased or decreased with anger and resentment. They felt that these variations were dependent upon the nature of the unconscious conflict rather than on current environmental stimuli. Engel et al. (1956) demonstrated increased hydrochloric acid production with outgoing emotional states, such as joy or anger, in an infant with a gastric fistula. The maximum level of gastric secretion occurred during states of anger, while production of hydrochloric acid decreased during depression and withdrawal states.

The experimental investigation of the relationship between emotional stress and colon function has been less extensive than that relating to gastric function. In an attempt to establish this relationship, Almy (1951) used proctoscopic examination and kymographic recordings of the intraluminal pressure of the sigmoid colon. He noted that the changes in the motility of the sigmoid colon were related to unpleasant emotional states in normal subjects and in those with an irritable colon syndrome. He concluded that nonpropulsive hypermotility was associated with ill-concealed feelings of hostility and aggression, and hypomotility with feelings of dejection and hopelessness. The latter emotional state was also marked by wavelike increases in intestinal tone, causing increased peristalsis and, consequently, diarrhea.

Grace et al. (1951) used 4 patients with exteriorized segments of colon to study the relationship between emotional states and colonic functions. Two of the patients had normal colon exteriorized for distal lesion and the other 2 for ulcerative colitis. Observations were made of contractility, mucosal color and mucous secretion. Life situations marked by fear and dejection were associated with pallor and lack of contractile activity, and those marked by anger, resentment and hostility were associated with increases in contractility and mucosal vascularity. Sustained hyperfunction of the colon, with increased hyperemia and contractility, was associated with an increased fragility of the mucosa and a propensity toward easy ulceration and petechial formation. Using similar methods, Wener and Polansky (1950) studied 1 patient with ulcerative colitis and noted that pain, fear and anxiety were accompanied by mucosal pallor and hypomotility, while anger and resentment resulted in hyperemia and increased contractility. These studies have been criticized for their imprecise description of emotional and psychological states, but they remain virtually the only studies in which there was direct observation of the colon during changes in emotional state.

Peptic Ulcer in Children

Peptic ulcer, once considered a rarity in childhood, is now recognized as an important cause of morbidity in the population under 16 years of age. Advanced radiologic techniques and a better understanding of variable clinical patterns have improved the diagnosis of peptic ulcer in children. Tudor (1974) set up a childhood registry for peptic ulcer in 1959 to collect unpublished cases of ulcers in children. He has treated 168 children with peptic ulcer since 1959. Another 791 peptic ulcer cases reported to the registry included 694 duodenal ulcers and 97 gastric ulcers. In 209 cases, there was a family history of ulcers.

Clinical experience suggests that there may be a causal relationship between life stress and benign ulceration of the stomach duodenum. Studies of individuals in acute stressful situations indicate that some of these individuals develop acute ulceration of the stomach and duodenum (Brod, 1963; Sawrey et al., 1956). Cushing's ulcer, neurogenic ulcer and stress ulcer are clinical examples of this phenomenon. There has been much debate about the causes and pathogenesis of these ulcers, but no firm conclusions have been reached. Whether or not gastric acid plays a part in ulcer formation is also questioned. However, increased vagal tone and humoral mechanism (that can be blocked by adrenalectomy) appear to be important factors in producing gastric ulcers (Porter et al., 1958).

The relationship of chronic stress to peptic ulcer formation is less understood than is the case with acute stress. Attempts have been made to show experimentally that chronic psychological stress can change the amount of gastric secretion and motility. Wolf and Wolff (1943) showed that in states of hostility and resentment, there is increased gastric acid secretion, increased mucosal blood flow and increased gastric motor activity. Some studies (Kehoe and Ironside, 1963; Mahl, 1953) have demonstrated increased hydrochloric acid production in states of chronic anxiety.

There are several psychiatric studies of children with peptic ulcer (Taboroff and Brown, 1954; Chapman et al., 1956; Millar, 1965; Lipton et al., 1966). These studies provide evidence of significant emotional conflict in children with peptic ulcer but do not establish a causal relationship between the emotional conflict and the peptic ulcers.

A diagnosis of peptic ulcer is made when barium contrast radiographs of the upper gastrointestinal tract show a definite ulcerous crater in the stomach or duodenum. These ulcers may be classified as primary or secondary. Peptic ulcers are classified as secondary when an underlying disease or ingestion of a drug or toxic substance is known to be the cause of the ulcer. They are classified as primary when no such predisposing factors are known.

The psychological management of children with primary peptic ulcer includes psychotherapy with the child and parental counseling. Many of these children are high-strung, much like one or both of their parents. Psychotherapy is focused on helping the child learn to relax and to deal with life situations without experiencing excessive tension. High-achieving parents are counseled to lower their high expectations for their child without reducing the affection they give him.

Ulcerative Colitis

Ulcerative colitis is a chronic inflammatory disease of the large intestine, primarily the rectum and the distal colon. The inflammatory process is generally limited to the mucosa, rarely involves the submucosa and is generally continuous from distal to proximal colon. The mucous membrane of the large intestine becomes hyperemic and bleeds easily. Diarrhea with bleeding and abdominal pain are the most frequent symptoms. The clinical course is marked by periods of remission and long chronicity.

Many theories of ulcerative colitis have been proposed over the years, but none of them have yet been fully substantiated. Psychological factors are usually emphasized in the etiology of ulcerative colitis, but exactly how emotional factors affect the colonic mucosa is not known, though effects mediated via the autonomic nervous system have been postulated. Until recently, most of the evidence pointing to a psychological etiology was derived from retrospective and uncontrolled clinical studies. After a critical review of the earlier studies, Engel (1954a,b; 1955) concluded that there was a relationship between the occurrence of certain stressful life situations and the onset of ulcerative colitis. These stressful life situations—ranging from an unwanted pregnancy and death of a parent to entry into a new job or military service—had a common denominator, which Engel defined as "a real, a threatened, or a phantasized interruption of a key relationship." Recent studies using control groups have produced conflicting findings. Monk et al. (1970) made a survey of 158 patients with ulcerative colitis and 69 patients with regional enteritis, together with suitable controls. All subjects resided in the same large city. They found no difference in the frequency of a broad range of supposedly stressful events in the lives of these groups.

Personality studies of children with ulcerative colitis frequently reveal that these children are rigid, dependent, distrustful, unable to express hostility, depressed, inhibited and generally immature (Alexander, 1950; Langford, 1964). Studies of the families of such children indicate abnormal patterns of family interaction. The mothers are found to be domineering and manipulative persons who often present themselves to their children as martyrs (Arthur, 1963). Fathers are described as ineffectual, passive and dissatisfied men (Jackson and Yalom, 1966). These characteristics, however, are not unique and specific to families of children with ulcerative colitis and, consequently, do not shed light on the relationship between patterns of family interaction and the onset and course of ulcerative colitis.

Although the primary management of ulcerative colitis patients usually rests in the hands of surgeons, internists or pediatricians, psychiatrists become involved in the treatment of a fairly large proportion of these patients. The role of psychotherapy in the treatment of ulcerative colitis is not well defined. In a controlled study (O'Connor et al., 1964), 57 patients with ulcerative colitis were treated with analytically oriented psychotherapy over a 7-year period and were matched retrospectively with 57 untreated patients with ulcerative colitis of comparable age, sex and severity of disease. The 57 treated patients, however, were referred for psychosis, personality disorders or psychoneurosis, while the control group had a relatively lower incidence of psychiatric abnormalities. The mortality and the incidence of colectomy in the psychoanalytically treated group were the same as in the control group. At the end of 8 years, however, the clinical and psychological grading of the disease was slightly better in the treated group than in the control group.

Such studies do not adequately answer the question of whether all patients with ulcerative colitis would benefit from psychotherapy or from other types of psychological intervention. Psychotherapy does not usually cure ulcerative colitis, but it should be considered an important part of the total management. Many adjustment problems created by the chronicity of the disease may alone warrant psychological intervention.

Anorexia Nervosa

Since 1868 when Gull first described the self-induced aspects of anorexia nervosa, there has been much controversy concerning the etiology of this syndrome. Discussions of etiology took a new turn when in 1914 Simond (Jessner, 1960) discovered that pituitary deficiency was a cause of anorexia nervosa. In 1930 Ryle (Jessner, 1960) reminded clinicians to look for evidence of psychological trauma in these patients. At present, there is a renewed interest in finding contributory endocrine and neurophysiologic factors. This renewed interest is, in part, a reflection of an increase in the incidence of anorexia nervosa.

A prosperous economy and cultural emphasis on slimness appear to be essential for the development of anorexia nervosa. Since World War II, there has been an increased incidence of anorexia nervosa not only in the United States but also in Japan, primarily in professional families who have adopted Western cultural values and practices (Ishikawa, 1965).

Primary anorexia nervosa appears to be a rather distinct clinical syndrome. It occurs most commonly in females between the ages of 11 and 17 years. The essential criteria for diagnosis are changed attitudes toward food, eating and body image. These youngsters begin to diet, with the explicit intention of losing a few pounds to trim their figures, but they seem to lose sight of their original aim. The pursuit of thinness becomes an obsession. Vigorous exercise is added to dieting in order to accelerate weight loss. Many of these youngsters lie about their food intake and self-induce vomiting if forced to eat. They deny their illness and show no concern over even an advanced state of emaciation.

American culture is obsessed with slenderness, and early and extreme attempts at weight control are frequently overlooked. An early warning sign that a weight-control program is excessive and obsessive is the extreme dedication with which the program is adhered to. Another warning sign is increased social isolation coupled with moderate to severe weight loss.

Most patients with anorexia nervosa come from intact middle-class families. They are described by their parents as well adjusted, compliant and obedient prior to the illness. They are usually bright, high achievers, active and somewhat shy.

Innumerable psychodynamic formulations have been made for anorexia nervosa, including rejection through starvation of a wish to be pregnant and fantasies of oral impregnation, guilt over aggressive impulses toward an ambivalently regarded mother, compliant attempt to get close to mother through a regressive identification (becoming a dependent young child), attempt to establish autonomy and self-initiated behavior, passive hostile control of a family which has overinvested eating with cultural symbolism and attempt to control sexuality by self-starvation. Family studies reveal the existence of pathologic interactions among the members of these families, which they make every effort to conceal. There is usually a great deal of parental discord beneath a facade of marital harmony. Each parent may seek affection from their "perfect child," who may feel obligated to fulfill these parental demands. The illness may thus represent an effort to escape from overdemanding parents and to establish a sense of independence.

Primary anorexia nervosa should be distinguished from secondary anorexia nervosa, which may occur in other psychiatric disorders, such as schizophrenia and hysteria. Some schizophrenic adolescents stop eating because of delusions of being poisoned. If the onset of anorexia nervosa coincides with the beginning of an episode of acute schizophrenia, the diagnosis of schizophrenia may initially be missed because of the intensity of anorexic symptoms and the unwillingness of the adolescent to share his thoughts with the physician.

Differentiation of anorexia nervosa from panhypopituitarism is no longer difficult, since adrenocortical and thyroid functions are preserved in anorexia nervosa. Occasionally, anorexia nervosa may be confused with the superior mesenteric arterial syndrome, in which patients limit their food intake to control vomiting, bloating and eructation caused by the occlusion of the third part of the duodenum.

Treatment modalities have varied during the past few decades from a very passive, nondirective type of psychotherapy to a very active intervention to promote weight gain (Minuchin 1973). In recent years, therapeutic approaches have been combined to include behavior modification, individual psychotherapy and family therapy. It is generally agreed that in the early stages of the illness, individual therapy and/or family therapy alone may be sufficient to manage these patients, but in cases where patients have lost as much as 40% of their former body weight and continue to defend their emaciated appearance as "normal" and "not too thin," strict methods to promote weight gain are combined with other therapies.

When a physician sees a child in the early stages of anorexia nervosa, he should record the weight and height of the child on the growth curve chart and share this information with the child and the parents. The degree of weight loss and the acceptable weight for the child's age and height should be pointed out. The physician should spend sufficient time with the child and the family to assess family difficulties and the child's underlying motivation to lose weight. This type of assessment will help the physician decide whether to continue managing the child himself or to recommend a psychiatric consultation. In the majority of these cases, family problems are not obvious, as most of the parents are reluctant to talk about them. Knowledge of the past history of the child and the family must then be used to decide about the need for psychiatric consultation.

If the physician decides to continue managing the patient himself, he should ask the patient to return for a second visit a week later with a weight gain of at least 1 pound (or in some cases no further weight loss). Most youngsters have not complied with the physician's request at the time of the second visit and make all kinds of excuses for their lack of weight gain. The physician should tell the patient and the parents quite firmly that, if the weight loss continues, the patient will have to be hospitalized. A third visit is scheduled a week later, and if the weight loss continues, the patient is hospitalized.

Most parents at this early stage of the illness do not realize its gravity and may be uncooperative in following treatment recommendations. A psychiatrist should be consulted before hospitalization to coordinate various types of therapies. The initial task of the psychiatrist is to convince the patient and the parents that anorexia nervosa is a serious, life-threatening condition and that the illness becomes much harder to treat if the starvation continues. Hospitalization is aimed at helping the patient to gain weight and to receive the necessary psychological treatment.

In the hospital, the patient's weight is carefully monitored, and tube feeding or intravenous feeding is instituted as soon as the weight gain falls short of the desired amount. In a hospital ward, confusion frequently prevails with regard to the circumstances under which tube feeding should be initiated and maintained. Orders for tube feeding should thus be explicitly written and explained to the house staff and the nursing personnel. Anorexia nervosa patients are very capable of manipulation of other persons. They may eat just enough to fall short of the weight gain requirement. The criteria used to initiate tube feeding should thus be rigidly and consistently adhered to in order to avoid manipulation by the patient or other staff.

The patient is discharged from the hospital after reasonable eating habits are established and the weight continues to increase. Individual and family therapy is considered essential by most psychiatrists for the majority of these youngsters.

Recurrent Abdominal Pain

In a survey of 1,000 primary and secondary schoolchildren, Apley and Naish (1958) found that approximately 12% of the children between the ages of 3 and 14 suffered from recurrent abdominal pains (RAP). Apley estimates that 9–15% of the general pediatric population suffers from RAP. Peak incidence of RAP occurs between the ages of 8 and 13 years. The maximum age of onset for boys is 9 years, while almost 50% of the girls have an onset between 8 and 10 years.

Pain is periumbilical in at least 50% of the patients. In the remainder, it may occur in the lower abdomen or in the epigastrium. The pain is characterized as cramplike in 50–70% of the patients. In the rest, it is either dull or acutely spasmodic in character. The pain is mostly episodic, but a few children may experience continuous discomfort punctuated by acute episodes of cramplike pain.

Episodes of pain are frequently associated with the following symptoms: pallor, headache, nausea, vomiting, obstipation, dizziness, poor appetite, weight loss and low-grade fever. No consistent relationship has been demonstrated among the onset of pain and meals, type of food, bowel movements, position of the body, activity level or the time of day.

Past history is frequently positive for gastrointestinal disorders. Myers and Thaler (1971) reported an incidence of colic in infancy in 15% of their patients, while Liebman (1978) found an incidence of colic in infancy in 29% of his patients.

Liebman also reported toilet training difficulties in 19% and enuresis in 18% of his patients. Family history revealed a higher incidence of gastrointestinal symptoms, peptic ulcers and recurrent abdominal pain in various members of the family.

Extensive laboratory, radiologic, and surgical investigations have not revealed definitive etiologic factors. Stone and Barbero (1970) found that in 102 children with recurrent abdominal pain, radiologic study of the upper and lower gastrointestinal tract, examination of stools for ova, parasites and blood, urinalysis and complete blood count were all essentially normal. Proctoscopic examination revealed nonspecific findings. Seventy percent of the children were given an electroencephalogram. Of these, 7% showed epileptiform records, 14 and 6 per second spikes were found in 16%, and an excess of fast and slow activity was determined in 36%.

Similarly, Liebman (1978) found that complete blood count, urinalysis and sedimentation rates were normal in 119 children with RAP. Examinations of stool for ova and parasites and stool culture, performed in 89 patients, were all negative. Urine cultures from 57 patients, upper gastrointestinal series performed in 99 patients, barium enema in 52 patients and intravenous pyelography in 34 patients were all normal. Proctoscopy and rectal biopsy were done in 18 patients, with nonspecific findings. Electroencephalograms for 22 patients were noncontributory.

PSYCHOLOGICAL FACTORS.—Several authors have emphasized social and psychological factors in the etiology of recurrent abdominal pain. Apley and Naish (1958) observed that children with RAP were more high-strung, fussy, excitable, anxious, timid and apprehensive than children without RAP. In his sample of 119 children with RAP, Liebman (1978) found a significant, positive relationship between the onset of pain and such events as periods of excitement (in 34%), school-related stress (in 26%), being punished (in 20%) and a recurrent change in school or residence (in 9%). Liebman also found a high incidence of family problems. Marital discord (excessive arguments and violence), separation or divorce occurred in 39% of the families within the current year and in another 5% a year or more before the onset of RAP.

MANAGEMENT.—Most of these children are hospitalized for diagnostic work-up. If a thorough diagnostic work-up fails to reveal an organic cause, this information should be given to the child and the family. Further efforts are made to explore sources of stress for the child if they are not already clear. Psychiatric consultation may be necessary to clarify the need for psychological intervention.

The management of pain is carried out on a symptomatic basis with an infrequent use of antispasmodics.

Liebman (1978) suggests a treatment approach for practicing pediatricians that entails frequent office visits for both patient and parents (for brief counseling) and environmental changes as suggested by the diagnostic evaluation. This approach resulted in complete disappearance of symptoms in 19% (21 patients), significant improvement in 69% (78 patients), minimal improvement in 10% (11 patients) and no change in 3% (3 patients). Only 6 of the 119 children were referred to psychiatrists for treatment. This resulted in significant improvement in 5 children and minimal improvement in 1 child.

Cardiovascular System

PSYCHOPHYSIOLOGY.—Although the impact of emotions on cardiovascular processes and functions has long been recognized, there has been a reluctance to conclude that emotional stimuli play a significant role in the pathogenesis of clinical cardiovascular disease in man. The influence of acute stressful situations on cardiovascular functioning is well known (Chambers and Reiser, 1953). Acute stress or emotional upset can affect one or all of the parameters of the cardiovascular system, i.e., cardiac output, peripheral resistance and blood pressure. A vast amount of literature has accumulated on the impact of acute stimuli in animals, ranging from direct stimulation of various areas of the brain to the effects of a variety of types of classical conditioning procedures. Although the major mediating system of cardiovascular response appears to be the autonomic nervous system, there is evidence for the participation of renal mechanism, of adrenocortical as well as medullary secretions of vasopressin, and probably other central nervous system polypeptides and releasing factors (Weiner, 1970).

Clinical experience provides many examples of the acute effects of stress on the cardiovascular system in man. However, a number of partially controlled laboratory studies (Shapiro, 1960) using acute stressful stimuli demonstrate that there are many technical problems in evaluating the significance of cardiovascular changes and the potential of stress to cause cardiovascular disease. Simple stimuli, such as venipuncture and mental arithmetic, are capable of producing pressor responses and changes in the cardiac output or in peripheral resistance. Shapiro's studies also suggest that the hypertensive and prehypertensive or genetically targeted individual responds more intensively to environmental and behavioral stimuli than do normotensive subjects. The hemodynamic characteristics of the stress response may be stimulus bound or patient determined and are further compounded by the fact that the overall changes in peripheral resistance do not reflect what may be occurring in different organ systems (Brod, 1963).

The effects of chronic stress on the cardiovascular system in man have been difficult to evaluate because most observations are experiments of nature, which are obviously retrospective. Two frequently cited epidemiologic experiments are the development of hypertension in exposed individuals following the Texas City disaster (Ruskin et al., 1948) and the studies of combat troops in the desert (Graham, 1945). Other evidence for the effect of environmental and behavioral stimuli has come from epidemiologic investigations, which have shown a positive relationship between elevated blood pressure and a number of environmental variables, such as type of city dwelling or stressfulness of job.

Data from these studies have been critically reviewed by Gutman and Benson (1971), who point out that urban populations usually tend to have higher blood pressure and that standard of living, income, education and type of occupation are all associated with significant differences in blood pressure levels.

Many attempts have been made to produce hypertension in rats by exposing them to stress for long periods of time. Early studies used sounds of variable frequency, which did indeed induce hypertension in rats. This hypertension, however, lasted only as long as the stimulus was continued (Ferris et al., 1945). Recent studies have been more successful in inducing chronic hypertension. For example, Friedman and Dahl (1975) were able to produce a significant elevation of blood pressure in salt-sensitive rats by using a long-term adversive conflict situation. Experimental manipulations in monkeys (Forsyth, 1969) have produced long-term blood pressure elevations, which have been associated with cardiac pathology.

Taken together, the studies relating stress to blood pressure changes and hypertension justify the conclusion that stress and cardiovascular functions are intimately linked. The question that remains to be resolved is not whether chronic stress plays a role in hypertension but rather to what extent, under what conditions and in which individuals these factors are acting as important pressor stimuli.

Respiratory System

PSYCHOPHYSIOLOGY.—The respiratory center in the medulla is quite vulnerable to the influences of cortical and subcortical stimuli. The respiratory rate shifts readily in response to emotional stimuli, as is seen in the hyperventilation syndrome occurring during a state of anxiety. The bronchial airway is innervated by the sympathetic and the parasympathetic nervous systems. The tone of the smooth muscles surrounding the bronchial tubes is regulated by various physiologic mechanisms (mechanical, neural, chemical and hormonal), which vary according to the different physiologic needs of the body and which regulate the size of the bronchial tubes and the amount of air exchange. In normal individuals, the tone of the bronchial smooth muscles is little influenced by suggestion, hypnosis or various emotional states. Persons with asthma, however, seem to be quite sensitive to these stimuli. Several studies (Dekkar et al., 1957; Luparrello et al., 1968) have shown that many asthmatic individuals develop a significant bronchospasm in response to suggestion or stressful emotional stimuli.

Bronchial Asthma

A genetic predisposition to asthma has been documented but questioned (Falliers et al., 1971; Ratner and Silverman, 1953). Opinions also differ with respect to the nature of the inherited defect. Allergists believe that the predisposition to asthma resides in the hypersensitivity of the respiratory mucosa, which reacts to certain otherwise harmless substances called "allergens" with the formation of antibodies. Subsequent interaction between allergens and antibodies results in the freeing of chemical mediators (e.g., histamine, serotonin and acetylcholine) which provoke bronchoconstriction, swelling of mucosal cells and increased mucosal secretion. Other theories ascribe the inherited (or acquired) defect to the deficiency of β-adrenergic receptors (Szentivanyi, 1968), parasympathetic dominance (Widdicombe et al., 1962) and a depression of hypothalamic and adrenal medullary response to stress (Mathe and Knapp, 1971).

Emotional disturbances also have been implicated in the etiology of asthma (Knapp et al., 1970). Although some of the earlier investigators (Alexander, 1950; Deutsch, 1951; Dunbar, 1954) proclaimed that emotional disturbance resulting from early maternal rejection is the primary cause of asthma, these claims have not been substantiated by controlled studies. There is no question, however, that an asthmatic attack can be triggered by an emotional upset in asthmatic patients. The frequency of such attacks varies greatly, depending upon the emotional state of the patient.

Several follow-up studies (Buffum and Settipane, 1966; Rackemann and Edwards, 1952) indicate that 15–30% of asthmatic children continue having asthmatic attacks in spite of rigorous treatment with allergic hyposensitization and bronchodilators. These findings suggest that allergic etiology alonc cannot completely explain the persistence of asthma and suggest the possibility that psychological variables play a role in its chronicity. The studies of Purcell and Brady (1969), Block et al. (1964), McFadden et al. (1969) and others indicate that there is a subgroup of asthmatics, perhaps as high as 50%, who are suggestible, essentially nonallergic and in whom emotions rank high as precipitators of asthmatic attacks. This is the group which is likely to benefit from conjoint psychological management.

PSYCHIATRIC MANAGEMENT

Almost all modalities of psychiatric treatment have been tried on asthmatic patients, including psychoanalysis, hypnosis, individual psychotherapy, family therapy, group therapy, behavior modification and residential treatment. The results of most of these treatments are hard to evaluate because of methodological weaknesses or short follow-up spans.

Most asthmatic children are likely to benefit from participation in short-term discussion groups, which can be organized by a social worker or a trained nurse in the outpatient clinic. Discussions center on the dependency of the asthmatic child upon his parents, fears of acute asthma attacks and the role of anxiety in the precipitation or aggravation of these attacks.

The children are encouraged to take part in normal physical and social activities. Similar discussions are carried on with groups of parents on an infrequent basis.

A small number of children who are extremely dependent upon their parents, who appear very withdrawn, who take no part in group discussions and who are minimally involved in daily social and physical activities should be referred for formal psychotherapy (individual or family therapy).

Hypnotic relaxation is generally not successful with children, but they can be taught to relax as they feel an asthmatic attack coming on.

Long-term residential treatment is warranted for patients who require frequent hospitalization but who generally remain free of wheezing during their stay in the hospital after the subsidence of the initial attack.

One treatment strategy based on conditioning theory is Wolpe's approach (1958) of systematic desensitization of asthmatic response to multiple, conditioned stimuli. A list of possible physical and psychological precipitants obtained from the patient's history is presented in a graded manner during a state of relaxation. Such a list of possible precipitants is usually not available in children and is subject to change over time. Another difficulty with desensitization therapy is that the attention a child receives during an asthmatic attack reinforces the operant asthmatic response to an indeterminant number of internal stimuli. A more fruitful approach appears to be the use of counterconditioning principles. The asthmatic patient is trained through biofeedback conditioning to control bronchial constriction and to substitute bronchial dilatation when faced with conditioned stimuli which previously evoked an asthma attack.

Biofeedback conditioning is carried out in two phases. During the first phase, which lasts for 5 sessions, preliminary training is given to establish an initial link between the rewarded response (bronchodilatation) and whatever internal or visceral cues are available to the child for self-initiation of bronchodilatation. The child breathes into a peak flowmeter and tries to increase his expiratory peak flow by turning on the signal light (triggered by the meter), which is set at gradually increasing levels. The child is rewarded for increasing his peak flow rate by the signal light and by verbal praise. During the second phase of training, which lasts for 10 sessions, this conditioned link is utilized to help the child overcome the bronchial constriction which is induced experimentally through suggestion, hyperventilation, exercise and, as a last resort, with the help of medication (e.g., carbachol). After the 1st month and again after the 6th month, 5 sessions of refresher training are provided to reinforce the conditioned link. This type of conditioning treatment is still in an experimental stage of development and requires long-term follow-up studies to establish its effectiveness.

Headache

Pediatricians frequently encounter patients whose primary complaint is headache. Sillanpaa (1976) reported on the incidence of headache in 4,825 Finnish children, age 7, who were beginning their primary schooling. He interviewed 87.8% of these children and their mothers regarding the occurrence of headache. The overall prevalence of headache was found to be 37.7%. In this group, 32.7% had occasional headaches (less than once a month), 6% had more frequent headaches (occurring once a month or more) and 3% had migraine headaches. These results were comparable with earlier studies, such as that of Bille (1962), who found an overall incidence of headache in 39% of the 9,000 Upsala schoolchildren in primary grades who constituted his sample.

Headaches are frequently classified into 3 broad groups (Diamond and Dalessio, 1978)—vascular, muscle contraction, and inflammatory and traction. Vascular headache includes migraine, cluster headache, toxic vascular headache and hypertensive headache. Common to all headaches in this group is a tendency to vascular dilatation which provokes the headache phase. The vascular dilatation is preceded in most cases, however, by vasoconstriction, which gives rise to prodromal symptoms, such as visual symptoms (blurred vision, dimness of vision or even loss of vision), transient hemianopia, ocular muscle paralysis and, occasionally, visual hallucinosis. Acute confusional state in toxic vascular headache refers to that state which is evoked by systemic vasodilatation and may be produced by fever, poisons, carbon dioxide retention and therapeutic agents, such as nitrates. Hypertensive headache is related to elevation in the systemic arterial blood pressure. Cluster headache rarely occurs in children.

Muscle contraction headache includes all types of tension headache resulting from chronic anxiety and depression. Inflammatory and traction headache includes headaches evoked by organic diseases of the skull or its compartments, including the brain, meninges, arteries, veins, eyes, ears, nose, teeth and paranasal sinuses. This group also includes headaches caused by mass-occupying lesions of the brain, such as tumors, abscesses and hematomas.

The pain experienced during a headache may originate from the cranial periosteum, the tissues covering the cranium or from certain intracranial structures. The intracranial structures that are sensitive to pain include the cerebral and dural arteries, the great venous sinuses and their venous tributaries from the surface of the brain, parts of the dural membrane at the base of the brain and certain nerves (trigeminal, glossopharyngeal, vagus and the first 3 cervical nerves). The structures which are generally insensitive to pain include the cranium, the brain, most of the dura, the pia-arachnoid, the choroid plexus and the ependymal linings of the ventricles.

Any rapid increase of pressure within the cranium will give rise to headache. The increase in pressure may result from a tumor, hematoma, abscess, edema of the brain or vascular dilatation. Intracranial vascular dilatation appears to be a significant contributing factor in migraine headaches. Lowering the pressure within the 3rd ventricle may also cause headache. This type of headache may result from withdrawing cerebrospinal fluid during a lumbar puncture.

The most common extracranial sources of headache are the pericranial muscles (contraction of which causes headache) and the extracranial arteries (distention of which causes headache).

PSYCHOLOGICAL FACTORS.—Psychological factors are commonly implicated in the etiology of migraine and muscle contraction headache. Dyken (1975) reports that migraine is the most common form of headache seen in children, but that it is frequently unrecognized and is confused with other types of headache. The etiology of migraine is not clearly understood. Many theories have been advanced, but none have yet been verified. Menkes (1974) found that children with migraine frequently were more angry than their peers without migraine but were unable (or forbidden) to express anger overtly. Ryan and Ryan (1978) report that these children are often shy, conscientious and strongly attached to their mothers. Various sources of tension that may contribute to the onset of a migraine attack include excessive excitement, school examinations, fatigue, family conflict and excessive parental or teachers' expectations for achievement. Riley (1937) noted that many of these children were completely free from their migraine headache attacks during vacations and believed that the tension and pressures of school contributed to the migraine attacks.

Muscle contraction headache is also very common in children. The pain is usually intense and diffuse but may be felt as a constricting band around the head. It may also be felt as a heavy weight on the top of the head, a dull continuous pain or an unpleasant feeling in the head. The pain may be generalized or localized in different parts of the head. The duration of the headache varies from a few hours to several days. This headache is frequently associated with spasm of the muscles of the back of the neck.

MANAGEMENT.—Migraine headache frequently requires treatment with such medications as phenobarbital, diphenylhydantoin, cyproheptadine and ergot. The ergot preparations, however, are rarely used to treat children. Muscle contraction headache is rarely treated with medication, with the exception of an occasional use of acetylsalicylic acid or acetaminophen. Anxiety or depression associated with headache should be treated with antianxiety drugs (e.g., diazepam or oxazepam) or antidepressant drugs (e.g., amitriptyline or nortriptyline).

In addition to medication, psychotherapy is generally considered essential for children with frequent tension headaches. The psychotherapy focuses on finding the sources of tension in the child's life. The child is then taught to deal with these tensions in ways that will reduce them. Modifying the child's environment (e.g., reducing pressure from teachers and parents) may help to reduce the level of tension. Sometimes parental or family counseling may be necessary to modify a tension-filled and chaotic home environment.

Breath-Holding in Babies

Breath-holding spells begin during the first 6 months of life and may continue until the child is 5 or 6 years old. Breath-holding usually occurs after a period of vigorous crying. When the baby suddenly stops breathing, he will first turn pale or blue and then become stiff and rigid. As the anoxia continues, the baby loses consciousness, and some babies may twitch or actually convulse. After losing consciousness, the baby no longer has voluntary control over his breathing, which thus resumes spontaneously, as does the return to normal coloration. The frequency of these episodes varies from an occasional occurrence to several episodes a day. These children are of average intelligence and have no specific physical problems. These episodes are sometimes difficult to differentiate from a seizure disorder, as some of these children may twitch or convulse while unconscious.

The exact etiology of breath-holding episodes is not known, though they are usually provoked by pain, fear and anger. Breath-holding often occurs after the child has suffered a painful injury or when the child is frightened or surprised. It also occurs during temper tantrums and vigorous crying spells.

These episodes frighten most parents (who worry about the possibility of brain damage) and often cause them to become both overprotective of their child and overpermissive for fear of provoking further temper tantrum/breath-holding incidents. Thus, the occurrence of breath-holding incidents has a great potential for modifying parent-child relationships and promoting behavior and personality problems in the child.

The management of breath-holding should include brief counseling sessions with the parents to help them understand the self-limiting nature of these episodes and their lack of any damaging effect on the brain.

REFERENCES

Alexander, F.: Psychosomatic Medicine: Its Principles and Applications (New York: W. W. Norton, 1950).

Almy, T. D.: Experimental studies on the irritable colon, Am. J. Med. 10:60, 1951.

Apley, J., and Naish, N.: Recurrent abdominal pains. A field survey of 1,000 school children, Arch. Dis. Child. 33:165, 1958.

Arthur, B.: Role perception of children with ulcerative colitis, Arch. Gen. Psychiatry 8:536, 1963.

Bille, B.: Migraine in school children, Acta Paediatr. Scand. 51:Suppl. 136, 1962.

Block, J. M., Jennings, P. M., Harvey, E., and Simpson, E.: Interaction between allergic potential and psychopathology in childhood asthma, Psychosom. Med. 26:307, 1964.

Brod, J.: Hemodynamic basis of acute pressor reactions and hypertension, Br. Heart J. 25:227, 1963.

Buffum, W. P., and Settipane, G.: Progress of asthma in childhood, America's Diseased Children 112:214, 1966.

Chambers, W., and Reiser, M. F.: Emotional stress in the precipitation of congestive heart failure, Psychosom. Med. 15:38, 1953.

Chapman, A. H., Loeb, D. G., and Young, J. B.: A psychosomatic study of five children with duodenal ulcer, J. Pediatr. 48:248, 1956.

Dekkar, E., Pelser, H. E., and Groen, J.: Conditioning as a cause of asthmatic attack, J. Psychosom. Res. 2:97, 1957.

Deutsch, F.: Thus speaks the body. Some psychosomatic aspects of the respiratory disorders: asthma, Acta Med. Orient 10:67, 1951.

Diamond, S., and Dalessio, D. J.: *The Practicing Physician's Approach to Headache* (Baltimore: Williams & Wilkins Co., 1978.)

Dunbar, F.: *Emotions and Bodily Changes* (New York: Columbia University Press, 1954).

Dyken, P. R.: Headache in children, Am. Fam. Physician 11:105, 1975.

Engel, G. L.: Studies of ulcerative colitis: I. Clinical data bearing on the nature of the somatic process, Psychosom. Med. 16:496, 1954a.

Engel, G. L.: Studies of ulcerative colitis. II. The nature of the somatic processes and adequacy of psychosomatic hypotheses, Am. J. Med. 16:416, 1954b.

Engel, G. L.: Studies of ulcerative colitis. III. The nature of the psychological processes, Am. J. Med. 19:231, 1955.

Engel, G. L., Reichsman, F., and Segal, H. L.: A study of an infant with a gastric fistula, Psychosom. Med. 18:374, 1956.

Falliers, C. J., Cardoso, R. R., Bane, H. N., et al.: Discordant allergic manifestations in monozygotic twins: genetic identity versus clinical, physiologic, and biochemical differences, J. Allergy 47:207, 1971.

Faulkner, W. B., Jr.: Objective esophageal changes due to psychic factors: An esophagoscopic study with report of 13 cases, Am. J. Med. Sci. 200:796, 1940.

Ferris, E. J., Yeakel, E. H., and Medoff, H. S.: Development of hypertension in emotional gray Norway rats after blasting, Am. J. Physiol. 144:331, 1945.

Forsyth, R.: Blood pressure responses to long-term avoidance schedule in restrained Rhesus monkey, Psychosom. Med. 31:300, 1969.

Friedman, R., and Dahl, L. K.: The effect of chronic conflict on the blood pressure of rats with a genetic susceptibility to experimental hypertension, Psychosom. Med. 37:402, 1975.

Grace, W. J., Wolf, S., and Wolff, H. G.: *The Human Colon* (New York: Hoeber-Harper, 1951).

Graham, J. D. P.: High blood pressure after battle, Lancet 1:239, 1945.

Gull, W. W.: The address on medicine, Lancet 2:171, 1868.

Gutman, M. C., and Benson, H.: Interaction of environmental factors and systemic arterial blood pressure, Medicine 50:543, 1971.

Ishikawa, K.: Uber die Eltern von Anorexia-nervosa Kranken, in Meyers and Feldmann (eds.): *Anorexia Nervosa,* Symposium am 24/25 April, 1965, Gottingen. (Stuttgart: Georg Thieme Verlag, 1965).

Jackson, D. D., and Yalom, I.: Family research on the problem of ulcerative colitis, Arch. Gen. Psychiatry 15:410, 1966.

Jessner, L., and Abse, D. W.: Regressive forces in anorexia nervosa, Br. J. Med. Psychol. 33:301, 1960.

Kehoe, M., and Ironside, W.: Studies on the experimental evocation of depressive responses using hypnosis. II. The influences of depressive responses upon the secretion of gastric acid, Psychosom. Med. 25:403, 1963.

Knapp, P., Mushatt, C., Nemetz, J., et al.: The context of reported asthma during psychoanalysis, Psychosom. Med. 32:167, 1970.

Langford, W. S.: The psychological aspects of ulcerative colitis, Clin. Proc. Children's Hosp. Wash. 30:89, 1964.

Liebman, W. M.: Recurrent abdominal pain in children: a retrospective survey of 119 patients, Clin. Pediatr. 17:149, 1978.

Lipton, E. L., Steinschneider, A., and Richmond, J. P.: Psychophysiological dlsorders of chlldren, Rev. Child Dev. Res. 2:169, 1966.

Luparrello, T., Lyons, H. A., Bleecker, E. R., and McFadden, E. R.: Influences of suggestions on airway reactivity in asthmatic subjects, Psychosom. Med. 30:819, 1968.

Mahl, G. F.: Physiological changes during chronic fear, Ann. N.Y. Acad. Sci. 56:240, 1953.

Mahl, G. F., and Brody, E. B.: Chronic anxiety symptomatology, experimental stress, and HCl secretion, Arch. Neurol. 71:314, 1954.

Malmo, R. B.: Activation, in Bachrach, A. J. (ed.): *Experimental Foundations of Clinical Psychology* (New York: Basic Books, 1962), p. 386.

Margolin, S. G., Orringer, D., Kaufman, M. R., Winkelstein, A., Hollander, F., Janowitz, H., Stein, A., and Levy, M. H.: Variations of gastric functions during conscious and unconscious conflict states, Proc. Assoc. Res. Nerv. Ment. Dis. 29:656, 1950.

Mathe, A. A., and Knapp, P.: Emotional and adrenal reaction to stress in bronchial asthma, Psychosom. Med. 33:323, 1971.

McFadden, E. R., Jr., Luparrello, T., Lyons, H. A., and Bleecker, E.: The mechanism of action of suggestion in the induction of acute asthma attacks, Psychosom. Med. 31:134, 1969.

Menkes, M. M.: Personality characteristics and family roles of children with migraine, Pediatrics 53:360, 1974.

Millar, T. P.: Peptic ulcer in children, Can. Psychiatr. Assoc. J. 10:43, 1965.

Minuchin, S., Baker, L., Liebman, R., et al.: Anorexia nervosa. Successful application of a family therapy approach abstracted, Pediatr. Res. 7:294, 1973.

Monk, M., Mendeloff, A. I., Siegel, C. C. I., et al.: An epidemiological study of ulcerative colitis and regional enteritis among adults in Baltimore, J. Chronic Dis. 22:565, 1970.

Myers, J. F., and Thaler, M. M.: Colic in low birth weight infants, Am. J. Dis. Child. 122:25, 1971.

O'Connor, J. F., Daniels, G., Flood, C., et al.: An evaluation of the effectiveness of psychotherapy in the treatment of ulcerative colitis, Ann. Intern. Med. 60:587, 1964.

Porter, R. W., Brady, J. V., Conrad, D. G., et al.: Some experimental observations on gastrointestinal lesions in behaviorally conditioned monkeys, Psychosom. Med. 20:379, 1958.

Purcell, K., and Brady, K.: The effect on asthma in children of experimental separation from the family, Psychosom. Med. 31:144, 1969.

Rackemann, R. M., and Edwards, M. C.: Asthma in children: a follow-up study of 688 patients after an interval of 20 years, N. Engl. J. Med. 246:815, 1952.

Ratner, B., and Silverman, D. E.: Critical analysis of heredity concept of allergy, J. Allergy 24:371, 1953.

Riley, H. A.: Migraine in children and the mechanism of the attack, Bull. Neurol. Inst. N. Y. 6:387, 1937.

Rubin, J., Nagler, R., Howard, M. S., and Pilot, M. L.: Measuring the effect of emotions on esophageal motility, Psychosom. Med. 24:170, 1962.

Ruskin, A., Beard, O. W., and Schaffer, R. L.: Blast hypertension: Elevated arterial blood pressure in victims of Texas City disaster, Am. J. Med. 4:228, 1948.

Ryan, R. E., Sr., and Ryan, R. E., Jr.: *Headache and Head Pain* (St. Louis: C. V. Mosby Co., 1978).

Sawrey, W. L., Conger, J. J., and Turrell, E. S.: An experimental investigation of the role of psychological factors in the production of gastric ulcers in rats, J. Comp. Physiol. Psychol. 49:457, 1956.

Shapiro, A. P.: Psychophysiologic mechanisms in hypertensive vascular disease, Ann. Intern. Med. 53:64, 1960.

Sillanpaa, M.: Prevalence of migraine and other headache in Finnish children starting school, Headache 15: [No. 4] 288, 1976.

Stone, R. T., and Barbero, G. J.: Recurrent abdominal pain in childhood, Pediatrics 45:732, 1970.

Szentivanyi, A.: The β-adrenergic theory of the atopic abnormality in bronchial asthma, J. Allergy 42:203, 1968.

Taboroff, L., and Brown, W.: A study of the personality patterns of children and adolescents with the peptic ulcer syndrome, Am. J. Orthopsychiatry 24:602, 1954.

Tudor, R. B.: Letter: Peptic ulcer in childhood, Lancet 2:219, 1974.

Weiner, H.: Psychosomatic Research in Essential Hypertension: Retrospect and Prospect, in Koster, M., Musaph, H., and Visser, P. (eds.): *Psychosomatics in Essential Hypertension* (Basel: S. Karger, 1970), pp. 58-116.

Wener, J., and Polansky, A.: Reaction of the human colon to naturally occurring and experimentally induced emotional states: observations through a transverse colostomy in a patient with ulcerative colitis, Gastroenterology 15:84, 1950.

Widdicombe, J. G., Kent, D. C., and Nadel, J. A.: Mechanism of bronchoconstriction during inhalation of dust, J. Appl. Physiol. 17:613, 1962.

Wolf, S., and Almy T. P.: Experimental observation in cardiospasm in man, Gastroenterology 13:401, 1949.

Wolf, S., and Wolff, H. G.: *Human Gastric Function* (New York: Oxford University Press, 1943).

Wolpe, J.: *Psychotherapy by Reciprocal Inhibition* (Stanford, Calif.: Stanford University Press, 1958).

4/Coping with Chronic Illness

DERRICK, an 8-year-old boy, has suffered from bronchial asthma since the age of 2 years. He was doing quite well, having only an occasional acute attack every few months. During the preceding 6 months, however, the frequency of acute asthmatic attacks has increased severalfold, to one attack of moderate to severe intensity almost every other week. He takes his medication conscientiously. His mother told the physician that she began working in an office 6 months ago for the first time in the last 10 years. She also reported increasing arguments with her husband during the last year.

Are some of Derrick's asthmatic attacks precipitated by acute emotional upset?

Julie is a 14-year-old diabetic girl. Her diabetes was discovered when she was 7 years old and had been under control until age 13. She was admitted to the hospital twice with severe diabetic acidosis during that year. Her mother indicated that Julie's personality has changed a great deal during the last year. She refuses to follow her diet, lies about food intake and even forgets to take her insulin. The parents feel that they are having difficulty communicating with her.

Is Julie's behavior due to commonly encountered lability of juvenile diabetes, or is it reflective of emotional difficulties?

Paul, a 15-year-old, heavily built hemophiliac, had been circumspect in his activities and sustained only an occasional injury. During the last year, however, he has been injured 5 times. His parents indicated that he has become aloof, stubborn and careless.

Is Paul denying the existence of his disease and unnecessarily endangering himself?

Jimmy, an 8-year-old boy, has suffered from epilepsy since age 4. His epilepsy has been well controlled with medication, and he has not had any seizures since the age of 5. During the last 8 months, however, he has had several grand mal seizures. In spite of higher doses of phenobarbital and Dilantin, he continues to have seizures. His parents separated a year ago, and since then Jimmy has become very difficult to care for, being frequently angry and throwing temper tantrums over small frustrations.

Is the recent worsening of Jimmy's epilepsy caused by his emotional upset over his parents' separation?

Case histories of children suffering from any type of chronic illness can be added to these few vignettes. Emotional problems not only influence the course of chronic illnesses but also cause problems in school achievement and social relationships. Sudden problems in these areas, when associated with a worsening of the medical condition, may be a sign of emotional problems influencing the disease process.

The prevalence of chronic illness in childhood is surprisingly common (Table 4–1). Of all children under 16 years of age, 7–10% are afflicted with chronic illnesses of a primarily physical origin (vital and health statistics 1976). The number of visits made by chronically ill children to a hospital outpatient department or to a pediatrician's office far outnumber the visits made by children with acute illness. A fair proportion of the pediatrician's time is spent not only treating the chronic disease process, but also managing acute crises and counseling parents on developmental issues, achievement problems, social relationships and vocational choices.

The influence of emotional problems upon a chronic disease may be quite apparent in some illnesses but completely obscure in others. For example, emotional problems are clearly present when a diabetic child is admitted with severe acidosis and we discover that he has not followed his diet or insulin injection schedule, or when a hemophiliac begins to deny his disease and to expose himself to injuries. However, the presence of emotional problems is not as demonstrable in cases of exacerbation of epilepsy or asthma. In order to understand the contribution of emotional

TABLE 4–1.—PREVALENCE OF CHRONIC CONDITIONS

DISEASE	RATE PER 1,000
Asthma	18.3
Epilepsy	9.3
Rheumatic heart disease	5.7
Severe retardation	3.6
Congenital heart disease	2.0
Deafness	2.0
Cerebral palsy	1.8
Cleft lip/palate	1.2
Mongolism	1.2
Legg-Perthes disease	1.0
Diabetes mellitus	0.8
Cystic fibrosis	0.4
Blindness	0.2

National Center for Health Statistics, 1976.

problems to the etiology of acute crisis during a chronic illness, it is important to understand the manner in which children deal with chronic illness.

Emotional Reaction of Children to Chronic Illness

A child's perception of his disease and his emotional reaction to pain, chronic discomfort or a handicap associated with a chronic illness vary with age, intelligence and the nature of the illness.

Preschool children utilize projection to explain the cause of their illness. They are likely to blame their parents or other significant adults for causing their disease. During the first 2 years of life, the child is still very dependent upon his parents. His needs for food and comfort are provided by the parents. When such a child suffers from pain or discomfort, he cannot understand why his parents cannot cure his discomfort. He blames them for letting it persist. His initial emotional reaction is anger, which is expressed as demanding and clinging behavior. If the parents do not understand the reason for the child's excessive clinging and demanding behavior and treat him harshly to snap him out of it, the child is likely to feel rejected and to withdraw in despair.

The development of the conscience or superego in early school-age children shifts the perception of etiology to the child himself. Children at this age are inclined to blame themselves for their illness and frequently interpret illness as a punishment for being bad. The understanding of cause-effect relationships is at a fairly concrete level during this age, and many children latch on to simple and frequently erroneous explanations of their disease. For example, a diabetic child reported that he had the disease because he ate too much candy, while a hemophiliac explained that he developed a hematoma because his "skin was too thin."

This type of emotional reaction to and perception of chronic illness continues throughout early childhood. As cognitive understanding of the disease is gradually acquired, however, simple and concrete explanations are replaced by a more valid understanding of etiology. Typically, the child's emotional reaction during these years fluctuates between getting angry at significant others (e.g., parents, siblings, doctors) and blaming himself.

By the beginning of puberty, the child usually understands the major causes of his chronic illness. His emotional reactions become more complex. He begins to ask questions such as "Why me?" He may feel sorry for himself and brood about his illness for days. Many parents try to answer such questions by telling the child how much better off he is when compared to other children suffering from the worst types of illnesses. Various philosophic and religious explanations may help some children to make the best of their handicap—"Life is not a matter of holding good cards, but playing a poor hand well," or "God gives hardship to those who can bear it."

While normal adolescents struggle to find an identity for themselves, handicapped adolescents have a much more difficult time in this regard. Feelings of inadequacy and of not being a complete or satisfactory human being dominate their thoughts. Their self-esteem, which is governed greatly by peer reinforcement during adolescence, also suffers some loss. Some of these adolescents, plagued by low self-esteem and confused identity, begin to deny their illness and begin to behave in irrational ways, e.g., the diabetic adolescent joining his peers in an all-night eating and drinking party or a hemophiliac getting into frequent fights.

This description of perception of an emotional reaction to illness is typical of children who were born with a handicap or who have suffered from a chronic illness since early infancy. Chronic diseases that begin in later childhood or adolescence cause varying degrees of regression of emotion and personality traits. The child may become more dependent on and demanding of his peers and friends. The regression may be limited to one aspect of daily life or may involve all areas, such as school achievement, social relations and personal habits. In older children and adolescents, withdrawal and a sad mood may prevail for months.

Body Image

Several authors (Horowitz, 1966; Linn, 1955; Loxley, 1972) have investigated the development of body image in handicapped children. Body image is defined as one's conceptual profile of his body. It consists of conscious and unconscious feelings, facts and perceptions about one's body. Head (1920) described the neurophysiologic concept of body image. The infant's gradual acquisition of body image is inferred from clinical observation of his increasing awareness of the parts of his body and their relationship with one another. The gradual development of neuromuscular control in normal infants depends on cerebral organization of the multitude of afferent impulses. The neurophysiologic body image may be considered as the frame of reference for the individual's interaction with the physical environment.

All types of emotional reactions are associated with the development of body image. The feelings associated with the body contact between the child and the parents and their verbal and nonverbal interaction become integrated into the child's body image. The manner of touching, holding and attending to the infant's needs conveys to him his parents' attitude toward his body. Approval and disapproval of his body or physical features are conveyed verbally as well as nonverbally. The child senses and imitates the parental attitude. Valuation or devaluation of one's own body reflects the value ascribed to it by significant others.

The formation of body image is a continuous process during growth and development. It is experienced at conscious and unconscious levels and is part of personal identity. Body image is also dynamic in nature—changeable in accordance with certain events (trauma, handicap, surgery) but only within certain boundaries. It tends to be quite stable throughout life. Phantom sensations following amputation are the most conspicuous and common example of the relative stability of the body image. Nevertheless, the perception of phantom sensations gradually disappears, demonstrating that body image may undergo modification and revision.

Children who acquire physical handicaps later in childhood usually undergo a lengthy and painful readjustment to the loss of their previously acquired functions. Such adjustment may be achieved through an acute mourning of the loss but is usually achieved only through a prolonged grief process which may continue for several years.

Factors Influencing Children's Adjustment to Chronic Illness

The conditions necessary for a child's good adjustment to chronic illness are realistic role definition and parental acceptance. Optimal adjustment requires that the child's role be clearly and realistically defined by the important authorities in his life (e.g., parents, teachers, peers) and that his parents value him, even when he is not playing his expected role with consistency. The difficulties encountered by handicapped children lie in the fact that they are confronted with more severe and more frequent adjustment problems than are normal children. Adjustment problems are exaggerated for handicapped children because their parents and other role definers often cannot furnish them with appropriate and unambiguous behavior standards for their new role and because cultural norms (from which few parents are immune) define any handicap as a loss of value or worth. The child with a handicapping condition is thus in limbo between two social worlds (Meyerson, 1958)—the world of the healthy child (with which his parents and other authorities are more familiar) and the world of the handicapped child (which is poorly defined and devalued). In fact, the handicapped child does indeed tend to see his role as somewhere between that of the healthy child and that of the sick child (Calhoun, 1967).

The following generalizations can be made about how the child will adjust to a chronic illness (Zachmeister, 1970):

1. The greater the amount of physical discomfort associated with a chronic illness, the poorer will be his adjustment. For example, regular

injections of medication will be more upsetting to the child than regular oral medication.

2. The greater the limitation of physical activity, the poorer will be the child's adjustment. A paraplegic child who is taught to use braces and crutches is likely to be better adjusted than the child skilled in the use of a wheelchair.

3. The greater the visibility of the handicapping condition, the less well adjusted the child will be. Cosmetic surgery done at an earlier age will lead to better adjustment (even if it must be repeated later) than cosmetic surgery done at a later age.

4. The greater the loss of sensory abilities (sight, hearing), the poorer will be the child's adjustment. A partially sighted child will have a better chance of adjusting to his disability than the totally blind child.

5. The later the age at which a chronic condition is diagnosed (or occurs), the poorer will be the child's adjustment. A congenital handicap will be adjusted to more easily than an acquired handicap of the same kind and severity.

6. The greater the amount of parental rejection (overindulgence or disinterest), the poorer will be the child's adjustment. Genetically transmitted illnesses produce greater guilt (and rejection or overprotection) in parents and, therefore, lead to poorer adjustment by the child. Increased support of parents of a handicapped child by the physician will increase the parents' acceptance of that child and thus improve the child's adjustment.

7. The larger the number of siblings younger than the chronically ill child, the poorer will be his adjustment. The parents of chronically ill children tend to have smaller families than parents without chronically ill children. Siblings younger than the handicapped child are likely to suffer more adjustment problems than siblings older than the handicapped child.

8. Severity of handicap interacts with family socioeconomic status: for middle- and upper-class families, the milder the degree of handicap, the poorer will be the child's adjustment, while for lower-class families, the milder the degree of handicap, the better the child's adjustment.

Parents of middle-class status are more likely to set unrealistically high goals for a mildly handicapped child than for a severely handicapped child, resulting in poorer adjustment for the mildly handicapped child. Lower-class parents tend to seek less medical attention for their handicapped children than do middle-class parents, resulting in poorer adjustment for handicapped children of lower-class parents, especially those with a severe handicap.

9. The less intelligent the child, the poorer will be his adjustment to a chronic illness. A child must have a minimum level of intelligence to adjust

to a loss of sensory ability, handicap or chronic illness. A more intelligent child is better able to understand his handicapped condition and, as a result, to have a more realistic self-image.

The above generalizations are based on clinical experience and a review of the literature in the area. They are not facts and should be regarded instead as hypotheses.

Coping and Adaptation to Chronic Illnesses

Coping with a chronic illness and a child's adaptation to such illness require that a chronically ill child receive all the social, psychological and emotional support possible. The child's own coping, or adjustment to the illness, taxes all his capacities and skills (Table 4–2). Improved coping demands that the child utilize his cognitive functions (such as perception, memory, speech, judgment, reality testing) to understand the meaning and cause of his illness. He should involve himself in motor activities as much as possible and express his emotions rather than withdrawing and isolating himself. At times, especially during acute episodes, use of denial and distortion help make the pain and suffering more bearable.

Well-adjusted Children

Several long-term follow-up studies of acute and chronic childhood disorders (Schulman, 1976) report a surprisingly adequate psychological adaptation on the part of children thus afflicted. The degree of overall adjustment is frequently assessed by and correlated with the level of achievement in school, the quality of peer relationships, the presence of activities, hobbies and interests, the positiveness of the self-image and the degree of self-satisfaction. The nature of certain handicaps may preclude the child's participation in some of these areas.

TABLE 4–2.—CHILD'S REACTION TO CHRONIC CONDITION

COGNITIVE RESPONSE	BEHAVIORAL RESPONSE
Child tries to understand why he is ill:	Fight—sees illness as challenge
Blames others—doctors, nurses, family	Flight—behaves as if nothing is the matter
Punishment—unjust	Surrender—feels defenseless against illness
Self-responsible	SOCIAL ATTITUDE RESPONSE
Not self-responsible	Conceals illness
EMOTIONAL RESPONSE	Becomes dependent
Anxiety, Anger } enemy attacking	Appreciates help
Depression—irreparable loss or damage	
Shame—concealment of illness	

Poorly Adjusted Children

Three patterns of maladjustment may be identified (Mattsson, 1972):

1. The first is characterized by the patients' fearfulness, inactivity, lack of outside interests and a marked dependency on their families, especially their mothers. They are passive-dependent, and their mothers are constantly worried about or overprotective of them.

2. The second pattern is shown by children who are overly independent and too daring and who engage in prohibited and risk-taking activities. Such children make strong use of denial of realistic dangers and fears. Many of these children have been raised by oversolicitous and guilt-ridden parents.

3. The third pattern may be seen in older children with congenital deformities and handicaps. They appear shy and lonely and harbor resentful and hostile attitudes toward normal persons who they feel should somehow compensate and repay them for their lifelong suffering. They usually are in families who emphasize their defectiveness and tend to isolate or hide them in an embarrassed fashion. They come to identify with their family's view of themselves and develop the self-image of a defective person.

Excessive sympathy of parents and others toward a chronically ill child creates an environment in which the child can manipulate and use his illness so as to satisfy his wishes and demands without developing his full potential.

Family Reactions and Coping

Faced with a diagnosis of a chronic illness in their child, the parents' initial emotional reaction is acute anxiety and fear over the possibly fatal nature of the disease. This initial parental anxiety interferes with their understanding and comprehension of all the diagnostic findings supplied to them by the physician. Denial and disbelief follow, especially if the child does not appear to be very sick. The parents may turn away from their physician on the pretext that he has not been sufficiently open with them or that he had not excluded other possible alternatives. They may consult several other doctors until they are no longer able to deny the reality of their child's condition.

A series of emotional reactions follows the acceptance of the diagnosis. These reactions include guilt, shame and mourning. The intensity of these emotional reactions depends a great deal on various aspects of the illness, such as age of onset, nature of the disease, whether congenital or acquired and the health status of the rest of the family.

Parental guilt arises from aspects of heredity, pregnancy, child care and religious beliefs. Many things can happen during pregnancy, delivery and early childhood that parents can construe as neglect, abuse or sheer misjudgment. Their search for possible causes and their desire to understand the meaning of their child's illness arouse all sorts of fantasies about heredity factors and religious influences. Parental guilt is very difficult to master and may continue for years if the disease is diagnosed as hereditary in origin.

Parents who are very insecure and feel inadequate about themselves are likely to feel shame in the presence of their handicapped child, especially if the handicap is obvious and visible. The awareness of such feelings perpetuates the parents' guilt. "What a monster I am! How can I hate such an unfortunate child who never asked to be born?" Ambivalent feelings of love and hate are also frequent, and most parents experience them in varying degrees.

Mourning and depression result from the realization of the chronicity of the illness. The intensity of the mourning will depend upon the value ascribed to the loss. A first-born handicapped boy in some families may mean a greater loss than in other families.

The better-adjusted parents do not excessively sympathize with or overprotect the handicapped child. Instead, they try to help the child develop his full potentials in social and educational areas.

Other members of the family, particularly siblings, may suffer from neglect and may resent the chronically sick child. One of the spouses (usually the father) may remain uninvolved for a long time on the pretext of being busy or unavailable. It is not uncommon for some of these parents to break up their marriage because one parent is overly involved while the other is completely uninvolved with the ill child.

Many families learn a great deal and mature from having a handicapped child. These families develop closer emotional ties with each other and function as a unit to face their difficult situation. They see their situation as a challenge. "Their lives become more significant, more basic, more meaningful" (Schulman, 1976).

Management

In practice, management of a chronic illness may be divided into three phases:

1. An initial phase when the diagnosis is made, the findings are communicated to the child and parents and treatment is begun to stabilize the disease.

2. A chronic phase during which the disease is stabilized and the child functions more or less normally.

3. Acute crises which occur during a chronic illness and which require special attention.

Initial Phase

Once the diagnosis of a chronic illness is made, it becomes the responsibility of the physician to help the parents and the child with the emotional crises that they suffer as a consequence of this revelation. The nature of the physician's relationship with the parents and the child is the most important factor in his ability to provide them with effective guidance. It is mandatory that the physician develop a relationship of mutual trust with the family during the initial phase; this makes for a better relationship later on.

In addition to building a relationship of mutual trust, the second most important factor in the physician's ability to help the family is absolute honesty. If the physician feels ignorant about any aspect of the illness, he should consult his colleagues or perform additional tests. There is no place for a quick diagnosis without complete work-up, since any incompletely investigated aspects of a chronic disease and any unanswered questions about it are likely to come up again in the course of the illness and will only lessen the parents' confidence in the physician.

Most patients experience a series of emotional reactions as described earlier. In most cases these feelings are resolved by themselves. There are some parents, however, whose denial and depression are so intense that they interfere with the adequate care of the child. Psychiatric consultation should be sought immediately for these parents. Some parents give an indication of denying the disease by their general attitude but seem to have no difficulty in adequately caring for their child. These parents need more time to work through their feelings.

How should the diagnostic findings be communicated to the parents and the child?

The ability to control anxiety in the face of bad news and the capacity to comprehend, at least cognitively, various aspects of the bad news vary a great deal among people. Most people are already so anxious when they visit a physician that they hear only selectively and retain very little information. The physician should learn to regulate his communication on the basis of manifest anxiety. Highly anxious parents and children need to be given diagnostic findings in small doses. A clearly written diagnostic report in layman's language is particularly helpful and can be handed to the parents after a postdiagnostic interview. A second appointment should be made in advance to clarify questions that may arise after the parents have calmed down and have had a chance to read the diagnostic report.

TABLE 4–3.—A PLAN FOR TOTAL CARE OF THE CHRONICALLY ILL CHILD

Thorough diagnostic work-up
Establishment of relationship based on
Absolute honesty
Mutual trust and confidence
Working through parents' reactions via
Direct counseling
Parents' organizations
Psychiatric consultations
Helping parents find support systems
Financial
Social—parents' groups, recreation
Directing parents' attention to spouse and healthy siblings
Child's care, requiring attention to
Organic aspect of the disease
Emotional adjustment
Education, rehabilitation, occupation
Social adjustment
Hospitalization—home care—office care
Dealing with acute crises

In summary (Table 4–3), the initial phase of management includes a complete medical work-up of the sick child, the building of a relationship of mutual trust with the family, recognizing the reality of the emotional crisis and guiding the parents and the child through a sequence of emotional reactions.

Chronic Phase

The chronic phase begins after the child is fairly well stabilized by the medical treatment. The focus of the management during this phase shifts from the disease to the total adjustment of the child and his family. Most children with chronic illness have adjustment problems in at least some areas of their life. Physicians need to evaluate various functions regularly by questioning the parents and the child. This evaluation may be divided into four major categories:

1. Organic condition, rehabilitation of the handicap
2. Emotional development
3. Intellectual and educational achievement
4. Social and economic areas

The treatment of a chronic condition should be simplified insofar as possible. Oral medications are preferred to injections if they can be taken by the child. The number of hospital and office visits should be minimized. If possible, parents, or preferably the child, should be taught to do exercises or tests rather than have them carried out by hospital personnel. If a persistent handicap is inevitable, emphasis should be placed on assets and abilities rather than on deficits and restrictions, e.g., does the child have a 20-degree limitation in extension or 160-degree preservation of function? The goal of medical care is maximum improvement of the handicapping condition and maximum development of compensatory skills, e.g., collecting hobbies for a child whose handicap precludes athletic success, lip reading for a deaf child. Both parents and children should be encouraged to read and learn about the disease to the limits of their understanding. They should be given opportunities to talk with the physician to clarify their confusion about certain aspects of the disease.

The physician should inquire about the emotional development of the child as well as the emotional adjustment of the parents. The presence of excessive anxiety, fear or depression in the family is indicative of poor adjustment. Similarly, an attitude of overprotection or rejection on the part of the parents reflects their difficulty in adjustment. The relationship between the parents and the existence of any problems with the siblings should also be explored.

Some handicapped children may be retarded and learning disabled. Physicians' guidance is necessary to advise the parents or to refer them to sources that can help them to find appropriate educational facilities for the child.

Chronically ill or handicapped children frequently suffer from social isolation and lack of peer contact. If the handicap is not too severe, the child should be encouraged to socialize with normal peers. Parents' groups and organizations relating to various chronic diseases and handicaps exist in most cities. The parents can be encouraged to contact these groups.

The economic burden of chronic illness is enormous. Most parents find themselves in a constant battle with health insurance companies and hospitals over the payment of medical bills. These parents need a great deal of assistance in finding financial support for their sick child.

Acute Crises

The occurrence of acute crises during a chronic illness always causes some regression and adjustment problems in children. These problems continue for a time even after the child recovers from the acute crisis until a new level of adjustment is attained. Each crisis presents problems similar to those described in the acute phase, although greatly scaled down. One parent remarked, "I was just getting organized and beginning to adjust my life around his illness, then all of a sudden this bombshell dropped." The parents and child both need extra support to get them through these crises.

Team Concept

As the sophistication of medical diagnosis and treatment has increased, so has the awareness of the multiplicity of problems that often exist within the same chronically ill individual. With increased knowledge, however, has come the need for narrower specialization, a wider variety of specialists and a concomitant loss of an integrative approach to the complexities of a single individual's diagnosis and treatment. Children with multiple problems may require the help of a number of different specialists who are jointly responsible for their care.

REFERENCES

Calhoun, S. H.: Self-concept and Stereotype in Chronically Ill and Healthy Children (Northwestern University; Master's Thesis, 1967).

Head, H.: *Studies in Neurology* (London: Oxford University Press, 1920).

Horowitz, M. J.: Body image, Arch. Gen. Psychiatry 14:456, 1966.

Linn, L.: Some developmental aspects of the body image, Int. J. Psychoanal. 36:36, 1955.

Loxley, A. K.: The emotional toll of crippling deformity, Am. J. Nurs. 72:1839, 1972.

Mattsson, A.: Long-term physical illness in childhood: A challenge to psychosocial adaptation, Pediatrics 50:801, 1972.

Meyerson, L.: Psychological aspects of sensory disability, Ann. N. Y. Acad. of Sci. 74:128, 1958.

Schulman, J. L.: *Coping with Tragedy; Successfully Facing the Problem of a Seriously Ill Child* (Chicago: Follett Publishing Co., 1976).

Vital and Health Statistics, 1976. U. S. Department of Health, Education, and Welfare. Superintendent of Documents. (Washington, D. C.: U.S. Government Printing Office).

Zachmeister, C.: Services for Chronically Ill Children. Unpublished paper, 1970.

5/Acute Anxiety and Fears

ANXIETY IS AN EMOTION accompanied by an awareness of its presence, certain physiologic events (mostly autonomic) and some outward behavioral manifestations. These 3 components of anxiety are not necessarily present at all times, and there are great individual variations in their manifestation. The emotional responses of a newborn infant do not include all the components. Some aspects of anxiety require the maturation of necessary structures before they can manifest themselves. Watson (1917) identified 3 inherited patterns of emotional expression in 6-month-old infants. Pattern X, tentatively identified as "fear," consisted of withdrawal responses and wailing cries in response to either a loud noise or a sudden loss of support (falling). Pattern Y, assumed to be "rage," was aroused by restraining an infant's movements, which resulted in strident crying and a flushed face. Pattern Z, called "lust," was caused by stroking of the skin, especially near the genitals and was accompanied by gurgling, smiling and sometimes by a penile erection. These emotions become further differentiated, and more subtle emotions emerge as the child grows older, e.g., delight, distress, rage, fear and jealousy.

In adolescents and adults, anxiety is differentiated from normal objective fear in the following ways:

1. Anxiety is diffuse or free floating and not focused upon definite situations or objects.
2. Anxiety is rarely accompanied by any degree of insight into its immediate cause.
3. Anxiety is prompted by anticipation of future threats against which current avoidance responses are not effective.
4. Anxiety is not controlled by any specific psychological defense mechanism, as are other neurotic reactions.
5. Anxiety is frequently expressed by somatic symptoms which may not be recognized as manifestations of anxiety and which may compel an individual to seek medical help.

Physical Manifestations of Anxiety

All bodily systems may be involved to varying degrees in manifestations of anxiety. Some individuals, however, appear to be more sensitive and aware of dysfunction in one or more bodily organs and frequently respond to anxiety-producing situations by experiencing dysfunction in that organ. The following somatic symptoms are common manifestations of anxiety:

1. Rapid and forceful beating of the heart, which may be accompanied by chest pain in the precordial area, whose intensity is unrelated to physical exertion or relaxation
2. Air hunger and hyperventilation
3. Dizziness, light-headedness and faintness
4. Flushing of the face, cold perspiration, goose bumps
5. Gastrointestinal symptoms, such as epigastric pain and the familiar sensation of butterflies in the stomach
6. General restlessness and frequent sighing

Anxiety is also associated with increased plasma levels of cortisol and free fatty acids.

Predisposition to Anxiety

Neurotic individuals show higher indices of anxiety than do nonneurotics in the areas of autonomic and endocrine functions. Anxiety-prone persons, who may be characterized as overreactors, have been estimated to make up between 5% and 10% of the general population. This estimate includes the small percentage of children who respond to the challenges of ordinary life (birth of siblings, illness, hospitalization) with anxiety and regression rather than with growth and maturation.

Tennes et al. (1977) studied the effects of psychological stress upon the level of cortisol excretion in 20 1-year-old infants. The stress imposed was a separation of the infant from the mother for 1 hour. The infants responded to this separation on a continuum from indifference to intense crying. The amount of cortisol secreted during a 2-hour interval after the separation was linearly related to the degree of manifest anxiety. An exception to this correlation were 2 infants who had low levels of cortisol and high levels of anxiety (as manifested by regressive withdrawal). The results suggest that constitutional differences are implicated in endocrinologic responses.

In addition to a biologic predisposition to anxiety, there are many environmental conditions—inconsistencies in relationship, poor management of stranger and separation anxieties—which can sensitize young infants so that they experience greater degrees of anxiety.

Mechanism of Anxiety

Although several theories have been advanced to explain the mechanism of anxiety, 2 theories have been especially popular and have generated a great deal of research.

The James-Lange theory (1890) defines emotion as the perception of bodily changes such that afferent feedback from excited bodily organs and systems peripheral to the central nervous system (CNS) results in a subjective experience of fear or anxiety. The famous dictum that we do not run because we are afraid, we are afraid because we run, summarizes the central idea of this theory. For James, the visceral sensations are the most important ones in defining the emotion. The somatic sensations of running and the sympathetically aroused sensations of rapid heart beat, panting and sweating are added to the simple perception of the threatening stimulus. Adding the somatic sensations, like running, to the visceral sensations results in a feeling of fear. The stimulus is, therefore, feared after the reaction to it begins. An illustrative example: You are driving at high speed when another car suddenly pulls out in front of you, you react quickly to avoid it, and only after the incident is over do you begin to tremble, sweat and feel frightened.

The Cannon-Bard theory (1915) suggested that bodily changes were of little importance as determinants of emotional experience and that emotions could be experienced without the occurrence of bodily changes. Accordingly, anxiety originates in the CNS. The visceral and somatic components of anxiety are secondary to the arousal of the CNS.

Several biochemical changes in the body have been causally related to anxiety states: rise in serum lactate, increased urinary cortisol, and increased levels of free fatty acids in the serum. In 1967, Pitts and McClure presented data to support their hypothesis that anxiety states are causally related to the specific effects of elevated serum lactate. They proposed that this causal link between elevated serum lactate and manifestations of anxiety may underlie all instances of pathologic anxiety. They also proposed a specific mechanism whereby elevations in serum lactate cause a fall in ionized calcium at the surface of excitable membranes through lactate-calcium complexing and suggested that anxiety states occur when this fall in serum calcium takes place at such excitable membranes as nerve endings. Several other studies (Bonn et al., 1971; Grosz and Farmer, 1972), however, have found that alterations in acid-base balance and/or endogenous lactate elevation and/or fall in serum calcium are not themselves necessary or sufficient conditions for the development of anxiety states. These studies, however, still leave open the possibility of a special susceptibility to lactate in anxiety-prone persons.

Studies investigating the relationship of plasma lipids to the arousal of anxiety (Gottschalk et al., 1965; Stone et al., 1969) have demonstrated that anxiety scores, derived from a speech sample by a content analysis method, correlate positively with the average level of plasma-free fatty acids (FFA) and with the increase in FFA to experimental stimuli. An increase of plasma FFA in fasting human subjects appears to be a sensitive indicator of the secretion of primary and secondary catecholamines. Catecholamines secreted into the circulation in response to anxiety mobilize FFA from body fat depots. Thus, plasma FFA (in fasting subjects) can be used as an indirect measure of adrenergic secretion. Increasing plasma FFA (i.e., by eating food) does not in itself increase anxiety, but increasing the anxiety level does increase plasma FFA. Similarly, parenteral injection of epinephrine and norepinephrine does not necessarily evoke the subjective experience of anxiety.

Types of Anxiety

Anxiety has been classified on the basis of its physical manifestations and on the basis of its underlying etiologic factors. Anxiety can also be acute or chronic, normal or pathologic. Different theoretical positions, such as psychoanalytic or cognitive, have generated different classifications.

The following types of anxiety are commonly encountered in children:

1. Developmental anxiety: Several stages of normal development are characterized by specific types of anxiety, e.g., fear of strangers in infants, separation anxiety in adolescents, fear of death in the elderly.
2. Traumatic anxiety: This results from an unexpected fright that overwhelms the child's defenses.
3. Contagious anxiety: Anxiety communicated to the child by any neurotically fearful adult with whom the child is in close contact.
4. Conflict anxiety: This has an intrapsychic origin and is the most important source of neurotic anxiety. The conflict may result from strong desires which are forbidden by the parents or the society.

Origin of Anxiety

Learning theorists attribute anxiety to a conditioning process in which neutral stimuli have become associated with punishment, pain and fear. Anxiety is an inevitable by-product of socialization. In infancy, the child has little awareness of the behavior that society rewards and punishes. His behavior is governed by his own selfish needs, some of which are socially taboo and are denied or punished by the parents. Under these circumstances, the adaptive thing for the child to do is to inhibit the unacceptable behavior and thereby avoid punishment, and, inevitably, this is the child's solution. This solution, however, is not entirely satisfactory for several reasons:

1. It leaves the original need unsatisfied and results in the putting aside or repression of this need. Psychoanalysts view acute anxiety as symptomatic of repression.
2. The origin of much anxiety is to be found in incidents that occurred

before the child learned to talk. Punishment for soiling during toilet training, for infantile sexuality, for lapses of table manners and for early aggression all instill anxiety for behavior which bears no verbal label. In later life, such verbal labels are of great assistance in developing discriminations between taboo and nontaboo acts. In early childhood, however, anxiety may be conditioned to vague, poorly differentiated aspects of behavior. It is impossible for a child to make completely accurate discriminations to avoid all punishment.

3. Punishment is often dependent upon the inconsistent moods and perceptions of parents and others in control of the child's life, with the result that it is applied inconsistently, thus making it difficult for the child to discriminate between punished and unpunished behavior.

Children predisposed to anxiety by virtue of biologic factors are likely to suffer more during the normal process of socialization and may manifest many anxiety reactions during their childhood and adolescence.

Role of Anxiety

Anxiety may be conceived of as a drive that provides a motivational basis for adjustment, since it is experienced as unpleasant. It helps individuals to avoid forbidden and anxiety-provoking situations. In some learning situations, mild anxiety enhances achievement. High levels of anxiety, however, interfere with performance and achievement.

Resolution of Anxiety

Techniques which serve to reduce the level of a person's anxiety are called "coping mechanisms" or "defense mechanisms." Generally the term "coping mechanism" is applied to healthy, adaptive mechanisms that lessen the anxiety and help the person to adjust to the demands of his environment or his internal drives. They are characterized by an adjustment to the pressures of everyday life and crisis situations that is free of the severe repressions which would continuously hamper the performance and effectiveness of the individual in the personal and social spheres of his life. The term "defense mechanism" is usually applied to techniques of adaptation to stress which create a great deal of anxiety and abnormal adjustment. Defense mechanisms include repression, regression, rationalization, denial and projection. It is usually the extent to which these defense mechanisms are utilized that determines the degree of the individual's maladaptation to society. For example, an isolated area of denial may not incapacitate a person, but a massive denial may adversely affect all levels of functioning.

Anxiety seems to play a prominent role in the development of all other types of disturbed behavior, elements of which may be regarded as techniques for reducing or avoiding anxiety. Anxiety reaction may be the consequence of an inability of a person to manage his anxiety in any other form. Phobic reaction occurs when anxiety is displaced on some symbolic object or situation. Somatic symptoms may be manifestations of anxiety. Similarly, obsessive-compulsive rituals may be the manifestions of displaced anxiety. Anxiety may overwhelm a person to such a degree as to cause aimless activity or freezing. Continuous interaction with an overpowering and, at times, hostile environment exposes children to many sources of anxiety. With normal intellectual and emotional development, children become aware of the risks and hazards which cause them specific types of anxiety.

Developmental Anxiety

Each stage of normal development results in a new perception of the world and is fraught with new types of anxiety. In early infancy, recognition of and attachment to the mother lead to the development of stranger anxiety. Further awareness of the environment generates separation anxiety. Other well-recognized anxieties include castration anxiety and death anxiety.

Stranger Anxiety

This phenomenon in American children appears around the age of 8 months and gradually disappears by 1 year of age. An 8-month-old infant will cry when approached by a stranger, and the crying will stop if the stranger stays away or leaves. This reaction develops at a later age in infants who are retarded. In some cultures where infants are constantly carried around by their mothers, stranger anxiety appears earlier. However, the infant is less likely to show fear of strangers if he is sitting on his mother's lap than if he is sitting a few feet from her.

Separation Anxiety

The situation that elicits separation anxiety is different from the one that causes stranger anxiety. For example, a 12-month child is playing in the living room with some toys, he sees his mother go to the front door and leave, and, as the door closes, he begins to cry. A 5-month-old infant would typically not cry in this situation. Separation anxiety appears in American children at about 10–12 months of age and disappears gradually by 20–24 months of age.

Mishandling of stranger and separation anxiety may prolong the duration of anxiety and intensify it. Lack of recognition of normal separation anxiety by some mothers and forceful separation from their infants may cause a great deal of harm, including difficulties in toilet training and problems in other stages of development.

Death Anxiety

By the age of 8, children become aware of the occurrence of death and probably have experienced the death of some animal pets or a relative. Although a full comprehension of loss by death does not occur until pre-adolescent years, the 8-year-old does have a partial understanding of the permanency of death. Children begin to worry about the death of their parents and other close relatives at this age. This normal fear may at times be heightened by separation from a parent or complicated by the child's own aggressive wishes toward the parents.

Chronic Anxiety

There are many children who have a permanent attitude of apprehension and overreaction to almost every unexpected environmental situation. Such a child is timid and shy in most social situations. He may do well in school, especially with an understanding and empathetic teacher, but he falls apart under demands for better grades and academic performance. His peer and social relationships are generally few and poor. Chronic anxiety may result from sensitization to separation anxiety and inability of the child to cope with rejection and separation.

Other Anxiety States

Conditions like hyperthyroidism, hyperkinetic syndrome and breath-holding attacks may have some component of acute anxiety. Early onset and continued history of hyperkinesis of several years' duration associated with a short attention span, easy distractibility and emotional lability help distinguish the hyperkinetic syndrome from states of acute and chronic anxiety.

Hyperthyroidism rarely occurs before the age of 3 years. The child with hyperthyroidism appears restless and hyperactive and shows frequent mood changes. A history of weight loss and school failure may be present. The skin of the child is warm and moist. Tachycardia is present at rest and during sleep. Fine tremors are observed in outstretched hands. Thyroid enlargement, an audible bruit, exophthalmos and high pulse pressure may be present. Laboratory tests for thyroid functions (especially serum levels of T_3 and T_4) are helpful in making the diagnosis.

Breath-holding attacks in children may lead to anoxia, cyanosis and unconsciousness. These attacks usually indicate a conflict between the child's wish for self-assertion and the parents' demand for conformity. The conflict may result from the parents' difficulty in setting appropriate limits. In a small number of children, breath-holding episodes associated with unconsciousness and convulsions may be early indicators of seizure disorder, requiring further investigation and anticonvulsant therapy.

Anxiety Manifestations during Sleep

Sleep is generally regarded as a restorative process for the weary body and mind. Mental activities, however, continue during sleep, and the unresolved problems of the day find their way into the dreams and other nondream activities of the night. Children, like adults, express much of their unresolved anxiety and conflict through dreams. However, as the egos of children are much more fragile, their anxiety dreams frequently turn into nightmares.

Anxiety in children is enhanced by the darkness of the night and is expressed in their reluctance to go to sleep, wakefulness at night, restless sleep and nightmares. A brief discussion of the general pattern of children's sleep will be helpful in understanding the manifestations of anxiety during sleep.

Pattern of Sleep in Childhood

Neonates spend an average of 80% of their time asleep and 20% awake, while the average 1-year-old is awake as much of the time as asleep. The proportion of time spent in sleep decreases as the child grows older. The rhythm and depth of sleep also change rapidly during the 1st year. For the first 3 or 4 weeks, the average infant takes 7 or 8 short naps a day, but the number is reduced to between 2 and 4 longer periods of sleep by 6 weeks of age. Seventy percent of all babies sleep through the night by 3 months of age. Another 13% settle down by 6 months. About 10% of all babies do not sleep uninterruptedly at night during the 1st year. The factors which influence this settling down are unknown. Environmental factors, such as adequate mother-child relationships, appropriate feeding procedures and adequate stimulation of the infant, have been implicated. It is generally felt, however, that a great deal of settling down is the by-product of CNS maturation. Infants who have suffered some perinatal insult, such as anoxia, settle down later.

There are great individual differences in need for sleep, and any particular child's requirement may vary from time to time. Many factors influence the quality and quantity of sleep. During the earliest months, intestinal upsets and, later, wetness, bodily discomfort, noise or emotional factors may interfere with sound rest. The infant's need for sleep or rest seldom becomes intense, as he will ordinarily sleep as much as is necessary and wake when he is rested. Later, he will have to learn the culturally approved patterns of sleep and wakefulness.

The EEG record of sleep in adults can be divided into 5 stages of sleep: Stage I is typified by low-voltage, fast activity with mixed frequencies, Stage II by the presence of sleep spindles and K-complexes against a low-voltage background, Stages III and IV by varying degrees of slow, high-voltage activity, and Stage V, rapid eye movement (REM) sleep, by the occurrence of Stage I EEG, binocularly synchronous rapid eye movements, suppression of muscle tone, and accelerated respiratory and cardiac rates. Nonrapid eye movement sleep stages (I to IV) lack REMs and are accompanied by the presence of muscle tone and slow, regular, cardiac and respiratory rates. REM and non-REM sleep represent 2 distinct states of neurophysiologic activity. REM is highly activated, while non-REM is basal and highly regulated. They follow each other in a periodic fashion and together comprise the sleep cycle. A typical adult sleep cycle starts with Stage I and progresses to Stage IV, then shifts back to Stage III, II and a REM period. This completes 1 cycle, which is repeated approximately every 90 minutes. The REM phase is associated with dreaming, though some mental activity does occur during Stages I and II.

In the newborn infant, polygraphic recordings are not as readily classified into distinct sleep stages as in adults. Infant EEG scoring manuals recognize 3 stages of sleep: active REM sleep, quiet sleep and intermediate sleep. Whereas active REM sleep and quiet sleep may be precursors of adult REM and non-REM sleep respectively, intermediate sleep represents an immature state of poorly organized sleep, found predominantly in premature infants but also present in young term infants and in some abnormal infants.

Sleep stage proportions change with age. Intermediate sleep, predominant in the premature infant of 34 weeks' gestation, diminishes and most often disappears by 3 months of age. At term, active REM sleep occupies 45–50% of total sleep time, intermediate sleep occupies 10–15% and quiet sleep occupies 35–45%. With increasing age, quiet sleep increases and active REM sleep decreases until late childhood, when young adult normative levels are achieved (20% REM sleep and 80% non-REM).

The length of the sleep cycle also changes with age. The cycle of normal infants at term has a periodicity of 45 to 50 minutes. More immature infants have shorter cycles, and premature infants of less than 34 weeks' gestation do not demonstrate sleep cycling.

Disturbances of Sleep

Table 5–1 is helpful in distinguishing psychological sleep disorders from physiologic ones.

Although some of the disorders, such as bedwetting and sleep walking, are listed under the physiologic category, they may also be caused by psychological factors. Further discussion of sleep disorders will be limited to such acute conditions as nightmares and night terrors.

The exact age at which a child begins to dream is difficult to ascertain. Due to the lack of verbal capability and the lack of distinction between daytime reality and dreaming, it is rare to obtain a report of a dream from a child before the age of 2½ or 3 years.

The incidence of disturbing dreams in children is fairly common. Shaw (1970) found that at least 20% of 3-year-old boys and girls report one or more disturbing dreams. The frequency of disturbing dreams in childhood is highest around 10 years of age, when approximately 33% of normal boys and 47% of normal girls report one or more dreams. The frequency of disturbing dreams gradually decreases during adolescent years.

Nightmares are disturbing dreams. The anxiety from the disturbing dream may persist for a while after the child is awake. The child, after waking and becoming fully oriented, is usually able to give an account of the fearful content of the dream.

Nightmares should be distinguished from episodes of night terror. Night terror may occur for the first time between the ages of 2 and 3. It is rare after the age of 10. A child with night terror does not wake up from sleep but may sit up in bed and cry or scream. He looks dazed, is perspiring and agitated and cannot be calmed down by any amount of verbal assur-

TABLE 5–1.—SLEEP DISORDERS

PHYSIOLOGIC DISORDERS	PSYCHOLOGICAL DISORDERS
Disorders of arousal	Restless sleep
Night terror (pavor nocturnus)	Nightmares (disturbing dreams)
Sleep walking (somnambulism)	Wakefulness at night
Sleep talking (somniloquy)	Hypersomnia
Teeth grinding (bruxism)	
Bedwetting (nocturnal enuresis)	
Disorders of sleep	
Narcolepsy	

ance. The episode may last for several minutes. The child sleeps through the episode and has complete amnesia for its content and its occurrence.

Nightmares are fearful dreams associated with anxiety and conflict. Treatment includes investigation and reduction of the anxiety-provoking situations in the child's life. Night terrors do not respond to psychotherapy. However, episodes of night terror occur so infrequently that no treatment is necessary. Diazepam at bedtime is helpful if the occurrence is frequent.

Manifestations of Displaced Anxiety

Unresolved anxiety appears to be at the root of all neurotic behavior. Various types of neurotic behavior are consciously or unconsciously adopted by individuals to cope with their feelings of anxiety. Variations in choice of neurotic behavior depend upon the personality type and the past experiences of the individual. Conversion reactions, obsessive-compulsive reactions and various sleep disorders are common manifestations of displaced anxiety.

Conversion Reaction

Older children frequently express their anxiety and conflict with symptoms that are mediated by the sensory and motor nervous systems. Sensory symptoms, if present, may involve sensations of touch, pain, temperature, vision, hearing, taste and smell. These symptoms usually appear as isolated and independent phenomena. They may last for months or be of relatively brief duration (days), with sudden dramatic onset and equally abrupt cessation. Conversion symptoms of pain, numbness or hyperesthesia characteristically do not follow the course of regional distribution of a cutaneous nerve. The glove-and-stocking type distribution of numbness is more commonly encountered. The anesthesias are never associated with atrophy of the muscles and rarely with abnormal reflexes. Disturbances of vision or hearing, such as partial or total blindness or deafness, are occasionally encountered in children. Disturbances of smell and taste are frequently reported by adolescents and appear to be related to their anxiety over intimacy with the opposite sex.

Motor disturbances may include abnormalities of gait, paralysis, weakness, fatigue and abnormal movements.

HYSTERICAL GAIT.—Gait abnormalities caused by anxiety and conflict are commonly seen in children late in the 1st decade and early in the 2d decade. The clinical manifestations may suggest a monoplegia, paraplegia or hemiplegia. Examination of a cooperative patient while he or she is lying down usually reveals normal strength, tone and coordination. A variety of bizarre and variable gaits may be noted. Often the pattern is irregular and variable in the same child. The patient may utilize the limbs normally for brief periods of time. The associated anxiety may result in a tremor of the hands or legs while the patient stands or walks.

The patient with hysterical monoplegia or hemiplegia frequently does not elevate and circumduct the foot but drags it along the floor or pushes it ahead. In addition, the expected hyperactive tendon reflexes, positive toe signs and ankle clonus are missing. A child with both legs involved may remain completely bedridden and refuse to use crutches and normal toilet facilities.

Most of the swaying during Romberg testing is at or above the level of the hips, whereas children with psychological difficulties sway from the ankles and must spread their feet apart to maintain balance.

MOVEMENT DISORDERS.—Involuntary movements of various types (choreiform, dystonic, athetoid and tics) are the most common manifestations of anxiety in children. They should, however, be carefully differentiated from well-known clinical entities, such as Sydenham's chorea and dystonia musculorum deformans.

Movement disorders based on organic etiology are attributed to abnormalities in the structure and function of the basal ganglia and its associated structures. In some conditions, such as Huntington's chorea, neuropathologic abnormalities are regularly found in the basal ganglia. In others, such as Sydenham's chorea and dystonia musculorum deformans, structural abnormalities are not found consistently, but basal ganglia abnormalities are inferred.

CHOREA.—Choreiform movements consist of rapid, involuntary, nonrhythmic jerks of various parts of the body. They are frequently present both proximally and distally and often involve trunk and face.

Sometimes choreiform movements are severe enough to be immediately obvious, but, frequently, a careful search must be made to detect these movements. The movements occur first in one part of the body and then another. They are marked by their irregularity and their failure to occur repetitively at a single site.

Sydenham's chorea is the most common form of acquired chorea in childhood. It may have an acute onset or may manifest itself subacutely several weeks to several months after a streptococcal pharyngitis. Three prominent features of Sydenham's chorea are hyperkinetic movement disorder, emotional lability and hypotonia. The movements characteristically ripple from one part of the body to another and tend to be distal. The patient often appears nervous, with aimless twitching movements of the extremities, face and trunk. Emotional symptoms of lability, withdrawal and outbursts of crying may bring such a child to the attention of psychiatrists for the first time. Sometimes the onset is so insidious that parents are unable to pinpoint the time of onset and see the child's emotional difficulties as having had a gradual development.

The antistreptolysin O (ASO) titer is elevated in only 65% of patients with acquired chorea, who show no other signs of rheumatic fever. Other antibody titers that are longer lived and are of greater diagnostic help are the anti-DNAase B and the anti-NADase.

Symptoms of Sydenham's chorea may disappear within 6 months to a year. Recovery is frequently incomplete, however, particularly with regard to the emotional lability, which may persist for several years.

In addition to treatment for rheumatic manifestations, tranquilizers have been found helpful for nervous symptoms. Antianxiety agents, such as diazepam, should be tried first for a few days before major tranquilizers, such as haloperidol, are substituted.

DYSTONIA.—Dystonia is characterized by simultaneous contraction of agonist and antagonist muscle groups. The muscular contraction occurs prior to the onset of movement, causing tightening and stiffening of the affected portion of the limb. The tightening persists during the movement and after the movement has been completed, so that the position assumed at the end of the movement is maintained for several minutes. Dystonia is distinguishable from athetosis, which also involves muscle contraction prior to and during a movement, because in athetosis there is a smooth flow from one posture to another without sustained posturing of the limb.

Dystonia musculorum deformans is a genetic disorder, an autosomal recessive form, commonly seen in Jews, with the onset occurring between the ages of 6 and 14. An autosomal dominant form is more prevalent in the general population. The first symptoms may occur in the limbs or in the trunk. In the initial stages of the disease, these children may be brought to psychiatrists, who may mistakenly make a diagnosis of hysteria or anxiety. Dystonia has been treated with phenothiazines with beneficial results.

TICS.—Tic is probably the most common movement disorder in children. It consists of rapid stereotyped movements in areas of the face, neck and shoulder and is usually directed away from the midline. These movements occur irregularly and last less than a second or may occur repetitively for several minutes. Emotional stress and excitement increase the occurrence and frequency of tic. Tic usually occurs in primary school-age children but may begin in the preschool years. A mild, localized tic may disappear after a short time. However, it is not uncommon for tics to become integrated into the child's movement pattern and to continue for years.

Treatment includes antianxiety agents, such as diazepam, and psychotherapy. Psychotherapy is designed to explore the stressful situations that precipitate or prolong the tic and help the child cope with these situations in alternate ways.

Gilles de la Tourette's syndrome.—This syndrome usually begins between the ages of 2 and 13 years with ticlike movements of the face and head. These movements gradually progress to involve the limbs and other parts of the body. During progression, facial movements are accompanied by vocalizations, which initially take the form of grunts, snorts, throat clearing, barks or clucks. In about half of these patients, vocalization becomes more formed, and words are heard, usually stereotyped, explosive, coprolalic outbursts. Symptoms undergo remission and exacerbation and get worse with emotional stress. The clinical picture may be complicated by other psychiatric problems (which are not the cause of this syndrome). Boys acquire the syndrome more often than girls, the male/female ratio being 3:1 to 4:1. The neuropathology of the syndrome is unknown. The EEG in half the patients shows nonspecific irregularities or rhythmic slowing in the theta range.

Treatment with haloperidol has been found effective in controlling the tics. The drug may have to be continued for several years, with some drug-free intervals.

Children's Fears

Normal developmental fears.—Children experience fear of particular objects and situations at different ages. These fears are usually mild and of short duration. Preschool-age children fear certain tangible objects and immediate situations, e.g., strange objects, strange persons, loud noises and falling. During middle childhood, there is fear of imaginary creatures, darkness, being alone or abandoned and death. There appears to be a decline of fears among adolescents, especially with regard to personal safety.

Fears are expressed by children in both overt and disguised ways. Young children express fear mostly in overt ways by crying and clinging to adults. Disguised expressions of fear are more typical of older children and can be discerned in their behavior, play and dreams. Overconfident, resistive, rebellious and defiant behavior may be manifestations of a child's disguised fears. An illustrative case:

A 4½-year-old girl asked her mother to fetch a doll that had been left in a room which was separated by a hallway from the rest of the house. She kept insisting that her mother retrieve the doll even after the mother had suggested that she get it herself. The mother then suspected what the matter was and said, "I will hold the door while you get it." At this, the girl ran happily to the room and got the doll. The mother recalled that her daughter had been previously frightened by the slamming of the hallway door, and now, instead of admitting that she was afraid, the daughter was trying to command her mother.

Many factors play a role in the acquisition of developmental fears. Watson (1917) observed that loud noises and sudden displacement (loss of support) were 2 basic stimuli to which all infants reacted with some fear. According to the cognitive theory of child development, any sudden, intense, unexpected or novel stimulus or any condition that demands some kind of adaptation for which the organism is unprepared, will arouse fear. The fear response is also mediated by the physical condition of the individual and the setting in which the stimulus occurs, e.g., a loud noise may not arouse fear when the child is with a familiar adult. The conditioning theory of child development states that most fears are acquired as a result of association with traumatic or painful stimuli. These fears are later transferred to other stimuli and situations through the process of generalization, e.g., a child who is knocked down by a dog in an alley may avoid not only that dog and that alley but other dogs and alleys as well.

At first, children's fears arise in response to occurrences in their immediate environment. Later, as they acquire the ability to dwell upon their past and anticipate the future, their fears become focused upon distant dangers, what the future may bring and their own impulses.

Intellectual maturation helps youngsters to better understand their fears but, at the same time, may bring additional or other imaginary fears. A child who is precocious or advanced in his development may be afraid of things that do not disturb other children until they are older.

Differential fear responses associated with age were shown in a study (Jones, 1924) in which a large, active, harmless snake was set free in an enclosure with persons of various ages. Children up to age 2 showed no fear of the snake, children aged 3 and 4 tended to be cautious and were hesitant to approach and touch the snake, and explicit signs of fear were displayed more often after the age of 4 and were more pronounced in adults than in children.

Emotional maturation is accompanied by better control over autonomic responses or expressions of fear. Illness, weakness or physical disability increases susceptibility to fear. Children may become afraid of vicarious dangers through their exposure to the mass media, including newspaper stories, movies and radio and television programs.

Dealing With Fear

Most fears that appear during the various stages of normal development disappear with maturation. Some fears, however, require intervention when they outlast a developmental period—e.g., when a child continues to be afraid of strangers after the age of 2, when fears are misplaced—e.g., a child fleeing when there is no pursuer, when they curtail a child's efforts to adapt to the daily stresses of life or when they create loneliness in a child's life (for many fears are unshared and unsuspected).

Children normally handle fears by avoidance, mastery through play and with support from adults. Fears of monsters, darkness, needles and bodily injury are frequently the themes of young children's play.

Holmes (1935) interviewed parents to find out how they handled the fears of their children. The following parental attitudes were regarded as probably doing more harm than good:

1. Consistently ignoring the child's fears
2. Ridiculing or punishing the child for being afraid
3. Forcing the child into the feared situation

The following methods were considered helpful:

1. Explaining the feared situation
2. Describing examples of fearlessness on the part of adults or other children
3. Positive conditioning—linking feared objects with pleasant stimuli
4. Successive approximation—gradually exposing the child to the feared situation

None of these techniques work all the time or in all cases because fears have many hidden aspects. Two children may say that they are afraid of dogs, but to one the dog may be a real dog on his street that is an actual menace, while to the other child the dog may be a figure of speech, for he is uneasy in the presence of any dog or at the thought of meeting a dog, even when repeated experiences show him that this or that dog is perfectly harmless. When he says he is afraid of dogs, he is telling the truth but not the whole truth, for he fears what the dog symbolizes rather than the external danger which the dog actually represents. The thing or situation feared by a child may represent both an external threat and an internal disturbance—this is especially true when children mention fears that have little or no basis in reality, as when a child says he is afraid of ghosts, or when a child with an excellent academic record says he is afraid he will fail.

Abnormal Fears

A phobia is an excessive and unreasonable fear of some object or situation. The phobic object or situation usually represents a displacement of the fear from the original stimulus that aroused it. The feared object is symbolically equated with the original stimulus. Lists have been compiled of the various phobias, the most common being fear of dirt, fear of high places and school phobia. Unfortunately, phobias tend to become generalized, so that a child who initially fears dirtying himself may end up avoiding a wide variety of objects in his surroundings.

SCHOOL PHOBIA.—School phobia is but one manifestation of a broad clinical category of school avoidance. There are many reasons why children may avoid school, such as a serious learning disability, fear of aggressive classmates or conflict with the teacher. School phobia is associated with intense anxiety that may result in prolonged absence from school. The anxiety may be accompanied by physical symptoms, such as aches and pains. If the child stays home, these symptoms usually disappear by noon or afternoon on school days.

Apprehension about starting kindergarten is a normal and generally transient reaction in young children. When, however, this fear persists for several weeks, school phobia should be suspected.

School phobia is more frequent in girls than in boys. There appears to be no relationship between school phobia and the child's intelligence, socioeconomic status or ethnic background. School phobia in children is associated with (1) an increase in mother's anxiety and (2) inadequate resolution of the child's early dependency on the mother. Many of these mothers also have an unresolved dependency need centering on their own mothers.

During early adolescence, school phobia may be precipitated by any situation that threatens the child's relationship with his mother, such as the birth of a sibling, mother's hospitalization, parental discord, child's own illness or a move to a new neighborhood. Unlike truant children who stay away from school to wander and play in the streets, phobic children refuse to go to school in order to stay home.

Therapeutic intervention should not be delayed once the nature of the difficulty is clarified. The child should be taken to school, preferably by both parents. The parents may have to spend some time in the school (at least initially) to support the child. The teacher and the principal should be informed of the child's difficulty and should help the child during this initial period. Sometimes a gradual resumption of school is best for extremely anxious and phobic children. The parents frequently require counseling to understand the contribution their own anxiety makes to the child's phobia.

Antianxiety medications, such as diazepam (Valium) or oxazepam (Serax), may reduce the child's anxiety and facilitate his return to school.

REFERENCES

Bonn, J. A., Harrison, J., and Rees, W. L.: Lactate-induced anxiety: Therapeutic applications, Br. J. Psychiatry 119:468, 1971.

Cannon, W. B.: *Bodily Changes in Pain, Hunger, Fear and Rage* (New York: Appleton, 1915).

Gottschalk, L. A., Cleghorn, J. M., Gleser, G. C., and Iacono, J. M.: Studies of relationships of emotions to plasma lipids, Psychosom. Med. 27:102, 1965.

Grosz, H. G., and Farmer, B. B.: Pitts' and McClures' lactate-anxiety study revisited, Br. J. Psychiatry 120:415, 1972.

Holmes, F. B.: An Experimental Study of the Fears of Young Children. in Jersild, A. T., and Holmes, F. B. (eds.): Children's Fears, Child Development Monographs 20:167, 1935.

James, W.: *The Principles of Psychology* (New York: Holt, 1890).

Jones, M. C.: The elimination of children's fears, J. Exp. Psychol. 7:382, 1924.

Pitts, F. N., and McClure, J. N.: Lactate metabolism in anxiety neurosis, N. Engl. J. Med. 277:1329, 1967.

Shaw, C. R.: *The Psychiatric Disorders of Childhood* (New York: Appleton-Century-Crofts, 1970).

Stone, W. N., Gleser, G. C., Gottschalk, L. A., and Iacono, J. M.: Stimulus, affect, and plasma fatty acid, Psychosom. Med. 31:331, 1969.

Tennes, K., Downey, K., and Vernadakis, A.: Urinary cortisol excretion rates and anxiety in normal 1-year-old infants, Psychosom. Med. 39:178, 1977.

Watson, J. B.: Emotional reactions and psychological experimentation, Am. J. Psychol. 28:163, 1917.

6/Aggression and Violence in Children

PEDIATRICIANS RARELY FACE direct aggression from a young child. Noisy protests, temper tantrums, occasional kicking or hitting is frequently provoked by painful and frightening medical procedures. Occasionally, a physician or a nurse may encounter a child who throws unprovoked temper tantrums and does not settle down in spite of repeated assurances from the doctor and the parents. In some of these cases, parents may reveal that similar temper tantrums occur at home and in school and ask the physician for advice. Early expressions of aggression in infants, such as headbanging, rocking, feeding difficulties, toilet training problems, self-directed aggression and hair pulling, frequently drive anxious parents to seek the advice of a pediatrician on what to do about them. Other aggressive activities of children, such as firesetting, destruction of property, harming other children and killing an animal, often arouse a great deal of parental fright, dismay and concern.

Scope of the Problem

All forms of aggression, including developmental aggression, reactive aggression, delinquency, firesetting, sadism, suicide and homicide, have increased in the juvenile population during the last decade. Suicide and homicide combined account for the highest number of deaths in adolescence. Crime statistics report only a part of the aggressiveness youngsters inflict upon people and property.

Crime index offenses include violent crimes, property crimes, murder, forcible rape, robbery, aggravated assault, burglary and larceny-theft. In 1978, more than 12 million index offenses were reported to law enforcement agencies in the United States. Estimated arrests for index crimes amounted to about 25% of the total reported cases. Persons under 18 years of age constituted approximately half of those arrested.

More than a million juvenile delinquency cases, excluding traffic offenses, were handled by juvenile courts in the United States in 1978. All areas, urban, semiurban and rural, have experienced a steep rise in these cases during the past decade.

Etiology

The causes of aggression are to be found in the biologic make-up of the child and its interaction with the environment. The contributions made by biology and the environment vary from individual to individual. Research on genetics, physique, temperament, endocrinology, brain damage and epilepsy have all contributed to a better understanding of aggression.

In 1953, Züblin found that men with the XXY chromosomal karyotype tended to exhibit antisocial behavior. Since then, a number of investigators have tested large groups of men for genetic abnormality and have found that although no more than 0.2% of male infants in the general population have an extra X chromosome, the XXY abnormality occurs more than 20 times as often as would be expected in male inmates of criminal and mental institutions. A recent international study of 46,150 newborn babies (Jacobs et al., 1974) showed that 1 in every 1,000 had the XXY or XYY chromosomal aberration. Although there are many XYY men who are perfectly normal, an individual born with XYY or XXY karyotype is statistically more likely to be incarcerated. People with an XYY pattern seem to have less ability to restrain themselves. They exhibit extremes of emotions, so that when they are happy they are excessively happy, and when they are angry and frustrated they are excessively angry and frustrated. Given the educational and social ramifications inherent in these genetic findings, a great deal more research will be necessary before designating these children as possessors of abnormal karyotypes.

Another area of investigation with relevance to aggression in children is of individual differences among newborn infants. There has been a steady increase in the number of studies concerned with the primary endowment with which infants are born. Organismic differences among the newborn may differentially determine the manner in which a child will deal with each maturational task. What may be involved here is not only an inherent difference in the unfolding of biologic functions but also differences in experiencing and perceiving universal childhood events.

In a longitudinal study of 136 children from birth, Thomas et al. (1963) grouped infants on the basis of certain reaction patterns. These reaction patterns, or temperament, referred to the behavioral style of the individual child and were assessed on the basis of the following variables: activity level, rhythmicity, adaptability, approach-withdrawal, intensity of reaction, quality of mood, sensory threshold, distractibility, persistence and attention span. The temperamental pattern most likely to lead to later behavioral problems was the combination of irregularity in biologic functions, predominantly negative (withdrawal) responses to new stimuli, nonadaptability or slow adaptibility to change, frequent negative mood and predominantly intense reaction. As infants, children with this pattern showed irregular sleep and feeding habits, slow acceptance of new foods, prolonged adjustment periods to new routines and frequent periods of loud crying. The mothers found them difficult to care for. These children later developed behavioral problems of an aggressive and delinquent nature.

Higher plasma testosterone levels in animals have been correlated with social dominance and aggressive behavior (Rose et al., 1971; Birch et al., 1945, 1948). However, a relationship between testosterone and aggressive behavior in humans is more controversial. Persky et al. (1971) showed that a group of normal young men reported significantly more aggression and feelings of hostility when their testosterone rate was high than when it was low. Kreuz and Rose (1972) found that plasma testosterone levels did not correlate with the incidence of fighting behavior in a young criminal population in prison but did positively correlate with a history of aggressive antisocial behavior early in life. Kling et al. (1973) found a positive correlation between plasma testosterone levels and individual aggression in psychiatric patients. Ehrenkranz et al. (1974) studied 36 subjects between the ages of 18 and 45, who were selected from the general inmate population of a correctional institute. They were divided into 3 groups of 12 inmates each. The subjects were selected on the basis of personal observations by the authors. There was a general consensus among several of the staff members that the subjects in group one were chronically aggressive; in group two, socially dominant without being physically aggressive; and in group three, nonaggressive. All subjects were given a battery of psychological tests, and blood samples were drawn to determine testosterone levels. The researchers found that there was a significantly higher level of plasma testosterone in the aggressive group as compared with the nonaggressive group or with the other two groups combined. The socially dominant group also had a significantly higher level of plasma testosterone than the nonaggressive group.

Brain damage of different types and degrees has been related to aggressive and violent behavior (Hertzig et al., 1969). Tumors located in the limbic structures of the brain can cause uncontrollable eruptions of violence, hostility and assaults. Malamud (1967) reported a study of 18 people with tumors of the limbic brain. All suffered from psychiatric disorders. Nine had tumors of the temporal lobe, and of this group, 2 were aggressive and assaultive, 2 were suicidal, 1 was both aggressive and suicidal, 1 had episodes of depression, 1 had episodic uncontrollable fear, and 2 others showed secondary psychotic symptoms. Patients with tumors of other parts of the limbic system were also described as being aggressive and assaultive.

Delgado and his associates (1968) have reported that all the behaviors characteristic of an aggressive episode, including violence and assault, can be produced by passing a weak electric current through the tip of a probe implanted in the amygdala. Furthermore, by varying the characteristics of the stimulating current and by changing the target area of the brain being stimulated, they could initiate and stop assaultive behavior.

Children with minimal brain dysfunction and hyperkinetic symptoms are generally more aggressive and violent than normal children. Studies of adolescents (Mendelson et al., 1971) who were diagnosed as having minimal brain dysfunction in childhood show that they exhibit more antisocial and aggressive behavior in their teenage years than do normal adolescents.

The major theories of aggression refer to it as: (1) instinctual, (2) a response to frustration and (3) an acquired drive. The most prominent theory of aggression is the instinctual origin theory of Freud (1955), who was impressed by the amount of destructive and aggressive behavior he observed in his patients and in the world around him. Many psychoanalysts reject his instinctual theory of aggression and suggest that aggressive behavior derives from other sources. Saul (1956) stressed unfortunate childhood experiences as the basic source of aggression. Horney (1945) suggested that aggressive behavior is one way in which a person can cope with basic anxiety. In both theories, aggression is regarded as a response rather than a drive.

Studies of animal behavior seem to support the instinctual origin theory of aggression. Dominance and fighting are widely observed phenomena in birds, mammals and some reptiles. But ethologists tend to explain such behavior in other ways: by attributing it, for example, to competition for food and sexual privileges or to territoriality. Significant correlations between dominance and fighting, age, sex, deprivation states, hormonal levels and neural structures have been reported.

Perhaps the most widely known theory of aggression as a reactive process is the frustration-aggression hypothesis. Aggression, however, is only one of a number of possible responses to frustration. Other responses may include regression and repression. Limited intellectual, physical or athletic potential may arouse a great deal of internal frustration. As a response to frustration, aggression is often viewed as a learned rather than an innate behavior, whose aim is the removal of obstacles to one's objectives. The frustration-aggression theory suggests that the control or reduction of violence requires reducing existing frustrations as well as constructive redirection of aggressive responses.

Learned aggression is presumed to result from aggressive childrearing practices and identification with or imitation of aggressive parents and significant others. Experiments on the effects of seeing films showing aggressive behavior have, with few exceptions, reported a stimulating effect on aggressive behavior. There are, however, several studies reporting a relationship between aggressive personality predispositions and a preference for aggressive content in pictorial media (Eron, 1963).

Responses of anger or rage are associated with aggression but need not entail the motivated infliction of injury. Anger does not necessarily involve destructiveness, whereas hate, violence and hostility do. In fact, anger has a strong communicative function for human beings and, therefore, has great constructive potential.

Aggression includes violence, hatred, hostility and all manifestations of destructiveness. Some authors (Rothenberg, 1971) believe that there are clear distinctions between anger and hostility and important distinctions between anger and rage, hate and violence.

Forms of Aggression

Aggression may be regarded as normal or abnormal. Normal aggression is exhibited by children during various stages of development. Another classification of aggression is based upon various manifestations of aggression, such as firesetting, sadism, murder, suicide, vandalism and cruelty to animals. A third classification is based upon the direction of aggression. It may be expressed directly at the persons who have aroused it, or it may be internalized and directed at one's own self, resulting in suicide or bodily injuries. It may also be displaced from the original object onto other objects, and, occasionally, it may be repressed and forgotten.

Developmental Aggression

Aggression is normally expressed by infants in two ways. The first is a rage reaction, accompanied by crying, motor activity and heightened autonomic functions, such as increased heart rate, blood pressure, respiration and reddening of the skin. The second way infants express aggression is by oral activities—sucking, chewing and biting. Although normal, these modes of expression may also be used by the infant to express aggression generated by frustration.

During the toilet training stage, the anal sphincter may be used to discharge aggression. Fenichel (1945) refers to the anal period as the "anal sadistic stage." There is an increase in verbal aggression between the ages of 2 and 4. One source of frustration for some young children is the necessity of sharing parental attention with other siblings. The birth of a new sibling may elicit expressions of aggression toward the new baby as well as toward the parents. The same dynamics also apply to sibling rivalry, which may generate a great deal of aggressive activity among the siblings.

During adolescence, fear, anxiety and insecurity frequently arouse disorganized aggression. Adolescents are unable to tolerate feelings of insecurity and weakness. They may go to great lengths and even severely endanger themselves just to prove their toughness. They may also hurt each other, not out of meanness, but to prove their indestructibility.

Biting, hair pulling, head banging and rocking normally occur to some degree in all children during infancy and the preschool years. There is, however, great variation among children as to the intensity and frequency of these behaviors. It is frequently hypothesized that maternal neglect is the cause of these behaviors. Infants require certain amounts of external stimulation for normal growth and development. This need is met by normal mother-child interaction. In cases of neglect, the infant is frustrated and tries to meet his stimulation needs through self-stimulation. It is not uncommon for some of these infants and young children to hurt themselves while performing their self-stimulating behaviors. Lourie (1949) studied a group of 130 children in a pediatric clinic population. He noted that 15–20% of the children had rocked and banged their heads in one form or another for varying periods of time. These manifestations usually began during the early months of infancy and frequently disappeared by $2\frac{1}{2}$ to 3 years of age. In some instances, these disorders are quite severe and may continue until the ages of 10 to 12 years.

Anger in its primitive form is a relatively undifferentiated response to hurt or frustration and is aimed diffusely and ineffectively at hurting or overcoming the frustrating agent—most often the parents. In preschool years, children frequently express anger by temper outbursts. By the time a child reaches school age, his anger is directed at specific targets.

An aggressive attitude on the part of parents may arouse abnormal or uncontrolled expressions of anger in their child and may delay development of impulse control. Overly submissive parents also inhibit the development of impulse control by giving in to the immature whims and demands of their children, who may, as a consequence, exhibit aggressive and violent behavior. Punitive parents use their children as targets for their own anger, often in the name of discipline. These parents frequently have marital difficulties and often come from homes where they were treated harshly as children. Rejecting and neglectful parents arouse anger and hostile feelings in their children. However, fear of being rejected prevents some children from directly expressing their anger. Such children may develop a storehouse of anger against life and people in general.

Firesetting

Firesetting is usually a symptom of a wide range of psychological disturbances but can also be found in normal children who go through a period of lighting matches.

Children in general are fascinated by fire. A match has magic qualities to a young child, since it can create light and warmth instantly. Most parents teach their children to avoid stoves and hot things. Some parents attempt to teach their infants a lesson by slightly burning their palms on a hot stove. In spite of these efforts, it is not uncommon to see some very determined 2-year-olds get burnt. Around the age of 5 to 6, when the child's motor coordination becomes good enough to ignite a match, a new interest in playing with matches develops. Witnessing this new interest, parents supervise the use of matches, allowing their child to light a candle for a family dinner or to start a fire in the fireplace, emphasizing at the same time the dangers of uncontrolled fire. Most children learn and abide by these restrictions easily. Only a few children continue playing with matches in dark places and in their rooms. Usually these episodes are few in number, and children grow out of them as the novelty wanes and parents make matches less available to them.

Most cases of firesetting by young children are accidental, but in some cases symbolic expression or anger and hostility is clearly discernible. A 6-year-old boy who set a fire under his mother's bed was clearly angry at his mother for divorcing his father, of whom he was very fond. Similarly, another child started a fire to burn a gift received on his birthday from his hated uncle.

Yarnell (1940) studied 60 children between the ages of 6 and 15 years who had set fires in various locations, such as at home and at school. The fantasies these children had about fire revealed that fire represented a strong force which could give them power over adults and which was partly magic in nature. These fantasies do not play an important role in normal children, but in emotionally deprived children fire may become the most powerful magic weapon they can imagine.

Kaufman et al. (1961) studied 30 firesetting boys between the ages of 6 and 17 years. Eight of the children were diagnosed as "primary conduct disorders," 11 were borderline psychotic, and the other 11 were overtly psychotic. The majority of the children in this group were seriously disturbed and had not advanced much in most areas of personality development.

Sadism

Sadism may be defined as pleasurable violence. Sadistic acts often have a playful character and have the same purpose as any other kind of play. Sadism as well as masochism are regarded as normal drives and are present in all children. Experiences of frustration during the oral, anal and phallic stages of development may increase the destructive element of sadism.

Cruelty to animals has been observed by Mead (1964) in a variety of cultures. She suggests that children who torture or kill "good animals" may commit more violent acts when they become adults. MacDonald (1963) reported that the triad of enuresis, firesetting and cruelty to animals is an unfavorable prognostic sign in those who threaten homicide. Hellman and Blackman (1965) studied a group of 84 prisoners, 31 of whom were charged with aggressive crimes against the person of others. Three fourths of this group had a history of the triad of enuresis, firesetting and cruelty to animals, whereas in the 53 subjects accused of nonaggressive crimes only 15 had a history of either the triad or part of the triad. Hellman postulated that the presence of the triad in a child may be predictive of later violent antisocial behavior.

Sadism related to sexual activity is rare in adolescents, although severe castration anxiety and aggressive threats may lead to sadistic attacks on the sexual partner. Fenichel (1945) believes that "sadists are fighting not only an unconscious anxiety over castration and over their own dangerous excitement but also contain self-destructive tendencies within themselves."

Homicide

Children possess the same emotions as adults and frequently act them out in their play. Most of these emotions, however, are unrefined, unrestricted and uncontrolled and are frequently expressed in extreme ways. For example, anger is expressed out of all proportion to the situation, and sadness may temporarily darken the whole world of the child. It is these extremes of emotion and their uninhibited nature that may lead one child to kill another. Such homicides include the newborn baby who is pushed out of the crib or dropped on the floor by a jealous sibling, or a game of cops and robbers that ends up in the inadvertent hanging of the robber. Lack of comprehension of the danger of firearms combined with extreme emotion also leads to many accidental deaths.

Denial of death and diminished fears for personal safety during adolescence lead to many accidental deaths in this age group. Most of the adolescents who commit homicide, however, are seriously emotionally disturbed. King (1975) studied 9 youths who had committed homicides. Their histories included violence in the home and inconsistent parenting. Their violence seemed to be related to serious deficits in cognitive skills, such as reading, language and general comprehension, with a consequent overreliance upon feeling. Unable to cope, they became alienated, reactive, violent and homicidal.

Malmquist (1971) studied 20 adolescents between the ages of 13 and 18 who were charged with murder. This retrospective study was designed to elicit the premonitory signs of homicidal aggression. A prodromal period of events was delineated before the homicidal act. The following events were highlighted by the study:

1. Behavioral change occurred shortly before the homicidal act (approximately within 48 hours). The most noticeable change was the development of deep pessimism about themselves or their predicament.
2. A call for help was often made by the youth, such as calling a hospital for admission or talking to a friend about the problem, but the gravity of the problem was rarely perceived by those in daily contact with the youth.
3. There was frequent use of drugs, such as barbiturates, other tranquilizers, amphetamines and marijuana.
4. Object losses that appeared related to homicide involved lovers and mothers.
5. Threats to manhood, often by teenage girlfriends, led to some of the homicides.
6. A buildup of agitation and energy, accompanied by motor restlessness and disturbed sleeping and eating patterns, preceded the homicidal act.
7. Homosexual threats, which arouse a great deal of anxiety in adolescents, caused some of the homicidal acts, primarily to escape or to punish the homosexual.

Halleck (1967) indicates that the final breaking point in individuals predisposed to homicide may be a feeling of helplessness and hopelessness, leading to an act of violence.

Episodic Dyscontrol Syndrome

There are millions of adults and children who become very aggressive and violent under the slightest provocation. These individuals have not learned to control their anger, and aggression becomes a way of life as well as a way to dominate others. There are some children in this large group, however, whose violent outbursts may be based on some type of brain dysfunction and temporal lobe epilepsy or some variant of it. Such children may be said to be exhibiting "episodic dyscontrol syndrome."

This syndrome is characterized by a storm of violence. Upon minimal or even no provocation, these children lose control, wreck property and act violently toward anyone in their way. Occasionally, the violence is directed against the self in the form of suicide or attempted suicide. The storm of violence may be preceded by an aura: a feeling of impending loss of control, a vague buzzing in the head, a jittery feeling or a nauseous feeling. Most of these children believe that something came over them to make them lose control. These attacks are experienced as alien, and the recollection of their content may be clouded. Some children dread the recurrence of the attack. Similar fears are often expressed by relatives who regard the episode as out of character with the rest of the personality.

Bach-y-Rita et al. (1971) studied 130 patients whose chief symptom was episodic violent behavior. On the basis of the chief symptom and the neurologic work-up, these patients were categorized into five groups. Group I (7 patients) consisted of patients previously diagnosed as temporal lobe epilepsy. Group II consisted of 30 patients with seizure-like outbursts, who lost contact with the environment during the outburst. Some of these patients experienced prodromal symptoms, such as aural or other stereotyped symptoms, including fatigue, depression, elation or sleep. Some also described an occasional amnesia, dizziness or an altered state of consciousness. Group III was composed of 57 patients with diffuse violence. Anxiety was very high in this group. Aggression was directed toward both animate and inanimate objects and sometimes toward the self. Group IV included 25 patients with a diagnosis of pathologic intoxication. These persons went wild after a few drinks. They usually had amnesia for the violent incident and appeared to be psychotic while they were out of control. The last group, group V, consisted of 11 patients with repetitive violence which was not associated with any altered state of consciousness.

Of the 30 patients in the second group, 15 received EEG examinations, and 9 of these revealed abnormalities—of the 9, 6 had EEGs compatible with a diagnosis of temporal lobe epilepsy.

Management

Psychological as well as pharmacologic therapies may be utilized in the management of violent children. Psychological therapies include family counseling, individual therapy and all the other types of social and environmental manipulations that may be necessary to provide a more suitable environment for the child.

The majority of aggressive and violent children will require intervention at the psychological level. There are, however, a small group of children whose violence is triggered more by organic dysfunction of the brain than by factors in their environment. These children, when recognized, are treatable, and their violence is preventable. Hyperkinetic and brain-damaged children whose violence is the result of their emotional lability, impulsivity and extreme excitability may be managed with stimulants (such as amphetamines, and methylphenidate) and sometimes with major tranquilizers (such as haloperidol, thioridazine, and thorazine).

Children with episodic dyscontrol syndrome should be given an extensive neurologic work-up to determine the presence of a possible organic etiology. Maletsky (1973) reported an 80% improvement in episodic dyscontrol syndrome patients treated with Dilantin (100 mg. 3 times daily). The lives of many of these individuals were changed for the better, and they became more able to control themselves. Their families no longer dreaded aggression.

Therapists providing psychological therapy to violent youngsters require a great deal of experience in dealing with them. The feelings of clinicians, teachers and other caretakers about violent youths are of primary importance in their care, therapy, education and rehabilitation. Feelings of both attraction and repulsion to the antisocial drives and behavior of these youths make it very difficult to find a reasonable therapeutic approach. Most people have negative and hostile feelings toward violent children, or they ignore the reality of violence in children. The psychoanalytic concept of countertransference provides a dynamic framework for cataloging feelings and recognizing their interplay in the child-caring, educative and clinical processes. This framework can be extended to the therapy of these youths, in that the acknowledgment and sharing of negative countertransference and counterfeelings, as well as realistic feelings evoked by the impact of a given situation, can be most beneficial in the treatment. In fact, there can be no treatment or education without this acknowledgment (King, 1976).

Some of these youths may not be able to function in society and will require institutionalization. Treatment programs, especially during the initial phases, are frequently very intense and reeducational and are geared to help the youths master social and cognitive skills.

REFERENCES

Bach-y-Rita, G., Lion, J. R., Climent, C. E., et al.: Episodic dyscontrol: A study of 130 violent patients, Am. J. Psychiatry 127:1473, 1971.

Birch, H. G., and Clark, G.: Hormonal modification of social behavior: The effect of sex-hormones administration on the social status of male-castrate chimpanzee, Psychosom. Med. 7:321, 1945.

Birch, H. G., and Clark, G.: Hormonal modification of social behavior. The effects of sex-hormones administered on the social dominance status of the female-castrate chimpanzee, Psychosom. Med. 8:320, 1948.

Delgado, I., Mark, V. H., Sweet, W. H., Ervin, F. R., et al.: Intracerebral radio stimulation and recording in completely free patient, J. Nerv. Ment. Dis. 147:328, 1968.

Ehrenkranz, J., Bliss, E., and Sheard, M.: Plasma testosterone: correlation with aggressive behavior and social dominance in man, Psychosom. Med. 36:467, 1974.

Eron, L.: Relationship of television viewing habits and aggressive behavior in children, J. Abnorm. Soc. Psychol. 67:193, 1963.

Fenichel, O.: *The Psychoanalytic Theory of Neurosis* (New York: W. W. Norton, 1945).

Freud, S.: Beyond the Pleasure Principle (1920), in Complete Psychological Works, Standard Edition (London: Hogarth Press, 1955, Vol. 18).

Halleck, S.: *Psychiatry and the Dilemmas of Crime* (New York: Harper and Row, 1967).
Hellman, D. S., and Blackman, N.: Enuresis, firesetting and cruelty to animals: a triad predictive of adult crime, Am. J. Psychiatry 122:1431, 1965.
Hertzig, M. E., Bortner, M., and Birch, H. G.: Neurologic findings in children educationally designated as "brain-damaged," Am. J. Orthopsychiatry 39:437, 1969.
Hope, K., Philip, A. E., and Loughran, J. M.: Psychological characteristics associated with XYY sex chromosome complement in a state mental hospital, Br. J. Psychiatry 113:495, 1967.
Horney, K.: *Our Inner Conflicts* (New York: W. W. Norton, 1945).
Hunter, H.: Chromatin-positive and XYY boys in approved schools, Lancet 1:816, 1968.
Jacobs, P. A., Melville, M., and Ratcliffe, S.: A cytogenic survey of 11,680 newborn infants, Ann. Hum. Genet. 37:359, 1974.
Kaufman, I., Heims, L. W., and Reiser, D. E.: A re-evaluation of the psychodynamics of firesetting, Am. J. Orthopsychiatry 31:123, 1961.
King, C. H.: The ego and the integration of violence in homicidal youth, Am. J. Orthopsychiatry 45:134, 1975.
King, C. H.: Counter-transference and counter-experience in the treatment of violence-prone youth, Am. J. Orthopsychiatry 46:43, 1976.
Kling, A.: Testosterone and Aggression. Paper presented at APA Annual Meeting, Hawaii, June, 1973.
Kreuz, L. E., and Rose, R. M.: Assessment of aggressive behavior and plasma testosterone in a young criminal population, Psychosom. Med. 34:331, 1972.
Lourie, R. S.: Role of rhythmic patterns in childhood, Am. J. Psychiatry 105:653, 1949.
MacDonald, J.: The threat to kill, Am. J. Psychiatry 120:125, 1963.
Malamud, N.: Psychiatric disorders with intracranial tumors of the limbic system, Arch. Neurol. 17:113, 1967.
Maletsky, B. M.: Treatable violence. Resident Staff Physician, pp. 40–44, Feb. 1973.
Malmquist, C. P.: Premonitory signs of homicidal aggression in juveniles, Am. J. Psychiatry 128:461, 1971.
Mead, M.: Cultural factors in the cause and prevention of pathological homicide. Bull. Menninger Clin. 28:11, 1964.
Mendelson, W., Johnson, N., and Stewart, M.: Hyperactive children as teenagers: A follow-up study, J. Nerv. Ment. Dis. 153:273, 1971.
Persky, H., Smith, K. D., and Basu, G. K.: Relation of psychologic measures of aggression and hostility to testosterone production in man, Psychosom. Med. 33:265, 1971.
Rose, R. M., Bernstein, I. S., and Holaday, J. W.: Plasma testosterone, dominance rank and aggressive behavior in a group of male rhesus monkeys, Nature 231:366, 1971.
Rothenberg, A.: On anger, Am. J. Psychiatry 128:454, 1971.
Saul, L. J.: *The Hostile Mind* (New York: Random House, 1956).
Thomas, A., et al.: *Behavioral Individuality in Early Childhood* (New York: University Press, 1963).
Yarnell, H.: Firesetting in children, Am. J. Orthopsychiatry 10:272, 1940.
Züblin, O.: Zur Psychologie des Klinefelter syndrome, Acta Endocrinol. 14:137, 1953.

7/Grief, Depression and Suicide

Grief

AT FIRST GLANCE, acute grief may not seem to be a medical or psychiatric problem but rather a normal reaction to a distressing situation. Early recognition of grief reaction may, however, help a clinician to avoid making a physical diagnosis on the basis of psychosomatic symptoms. Ordinary grief reaction should be distinguished from depression. Children and adolescents frequently experience losses of loved ones due to separation and death. The intensity and manner of expression of grief depend on the age of the child. Infants and young children express grief over separation of the parents through stages of protest, despair and detachment. When separated from their parents, young children under 3 years of age settle down into despair after a period of crying. It is not uncommon for parents to come home after a few days of vacation and find their young child detached and unresponsive, at least for a brief period of time. If the separation was a lengthy one, the child's detachment and withdrawal may continue for several days.

The duration and intensity of grief experienced by older children depend upon the nature of their relationship with the deceased and the degree to which they understand the finality of death. Three definable stages of grief are recognized by several studies (Parker, 1970; Lewis, 1961).

1. The first stage of grief consists of shock, numbness and disbelief. The news of somebody's death arouses a quick denial, which may last from a few minutes to several days. The defense mechanism of denial serves an adaptive function and helps the person to cope with the initial shock.

2. The second stage of grief includes painful longing and preoccupation with memories and mental images of the deceased person. This stage begins after the initial reaction of shock and may not reach its peak until the 2d to 4th week following the death. Once having peaked, these reactions gradually subside. Characteristic reactions are recurrent, wavelike experiences of tearful longing for the deceased person, associated with thoughts, memories and mental images of the person. These waves are often triggered by items or events associated with the deceased person. Through such recurrences of memory, the mourner says goodbye to the deceased person. These reactions are intense for about 3 months, then decline progressively over the following 6 to 12 months.

3. Stage three is one of resolution of grief and resumption of ordinary life activities, although the person continues to experience periodic episodes of sadness and painful longing.

Grief reaction may be delayed or expressed in a distorted fashion. The delay may occur when the person is confronted with other important tasks and is not able to afford the luxury of grief reactions. Distorted expressions of grief reaction include delinquency, stealing, lying and somatic symptoms.

Depression

The presence of a sustained state of depression in young children is a controversial issue in child psychiatry. Some of the controversy is generated by varying use of the term "depression." On the one hand, the presence of any sad, dysphoric or despondent mood is considered depression, while on the other hand, depression is regarded as a syndrome or clinical entity with a cluster of signs and symptoms. Most of the empirical studies of depression in children utilize an adult diagnostic model incorporating certain modifications (Feighner et al., 1972). For this reason, it may be helpful to review the clinical entity of depression as it occurs in adults.

Adult Depression

The *Diagnostic and Statistical Manual of Mental Disorders* (DSM-III, 1978) suggests classifying affective disorders into the following 3 broad groups which are further subdivided into several categories:

1. Episodic affective disorders
2. Chronic affective disorders
3. Atypical affective disorders

Episodic affective disorders are defined as acute episodes of illness (depressive or manic) when they are clearly distinguishable from prior functioning. This group is subdivided into unipolar and bipolar. The unipolar subgroup relates to the occurrence of only 1 affective disorder, either mania or depression, while the bipolar subgroup relates to the occurrence of alternating episodes of mania and depression. Acute depression episodes are classified as neurotic vs. psychotic, agitated vs. retarded and primary vs. secondary.

An acute manic episode is characterized by the presence of distinctly elated, expansive or irritable moods. The patient is usually more active than usual, more talkative, has flights of ideas, inflated self-esteem and decreased need of sleep, is highly distractible and engages in activities without regard for possible painful consequences.

An acute depressive episode is characterized by the presence of sustained depressed or sad mood, poor appetite, sleep disturbance (difficulty in sleeping or sleeping too much), loss of energy, fatigability or tiredness, loss of interest or pleasure in usual activities, feelings of self-reproach, excessive or inappropriate guilt, diminished ability to think or concentrate and recurrent thoughts of death or suicide.

A bipolar affective disorder episode is characterized by the full symptomatic picture of both manic and depressive episodes, intermixed or rapidly alternating every few days.

Chronic affective disorders are defined as long-standing (at least 2 years) illnesses which usually do not have a clearly distinguishable cause. Disturbances of mood may be sustained through the period of illness or may occur intermittently. Chronic affective disorders are subdivided into:

1. Chronic hypomanic disorder
2. Chronic depressive disorder
3. Cyclothymic disorder

A chronic hypomanic disorder involves an elevated, expansive or irritable mood and associated symptoms, which is not of sufficient severity to meet the criteria for acute manic episode. Other characteristic symptoms of acute manic episode, such as delusions and looseness of association, are absent.

A chronic depressive disorder involves depressed mood and loss of interest and pleasure in almost all activities, not of sufficient severity to meet the criteria for episodic depression.

A cyclothymic disorder involves characteristics of both hypomanic and depressive disorders, not severe enough to meet the criteria for manic or depressive episodes. In severe cases, manifestations of hypomania and depression may be separated by periods of a normal mood lasting several months. In other cases, the two syndromes are intermixed or alternate periodically.

Atypical affective disorders include atypical cases of manic or depressive disorders which cannot be classified according to previously discussed criteria.

Manic-depressive illness is regarded as a psychobiologic disease. Its manifestations are influenced by predisposing factors of heredity, constitution and development, and it is precipitated by an interaction of biologic and psychological factors. A great deal of research is being carried out to determine the degree to which these various factors contribute to this illness.

The worldwide incidence of manic-depressive illness is estimated to be about 3 to 4 per thousand. Studies of monozygotic and dyzygotic twins (Kallmann, 1953) indicate an incidence of manic-depressive illness of 20–25% in siblings and nonidentical twins.

Investigation of biologic factors relates primarily to disturbances in metabolism of catecholamines and steroids. Urinary excretion of epinephrine, norepinephrine and their precursors and metabolites are altered in patients with affective disorders. Similarly, changes in the metabolism of adrenal steroids have also been reported in depression.

Child Depression

Many rating scales have been designed to objectively assess the presence and severity of depression in adults. Some of these scales have been modified to assess depression in children (McConville et al., 1973; Weinberg et al., 1973; Connell, 1972; Renshaw, 1974). McConville and associates' list of characteristics of childhood depression included the following 15 items:

1. Sadness
2. Helplessness
3. Loneliness
4. Feelings of loss
5. Unspecified feelings of being bad
6. Negative self-esteem
7. Feelings of being unable to help
8. Unable to do things for others
9. Inability to be liked
10. Expectations of being used
11. Feelings that the situation will not change
12. Feelings of being wicked
13. Feelings of being hated because of actions
14. Feelings of being justly punished
15. Suicidal ideation

On the basis of some clustering of these items, the authors describe three types of childhood depression: (1) affectual depression—includes expression of sadness, helplessness and occasional hopelessness, (2) negative self-esteem depression—includes feelings of worthlessness, being unloved and being used by other people, (3) guilt depression—occurs in a small group of children who feel that they are wicked and that they should be punished or killed.

Glaser (1968) asserts that childhood depression is a different entity than the depression of adults. He takes the position that childhood depression is generally masked and is not readily identifiable by the presenting symptoms. Several other authors (Toolan, 1962; Cytryn and McKnew, 1974) concur. Masked depression is expressed by a variety of symptoms that are regarded as depressive equivalents, such as delinquent behavior, psychoneurotic reactions and psychophysiologic reactions. Table 7-1 lists the

TABLE 7–1.—MASKED SYMPTOMS OF DEPRESSION IN CHILDREN

GLASER, 1968	TOOLAN, 1962	CYTRYN AND McKNEW, 1974
1. Temper tantrums, disobedience, truancy, running away, delinquent behavior	1. Temper tantrums	1. Hyperactivity
2. School phobia, failure to achieve in school, other psychoneurotic reactions	2. Disobedience	2. Aggressiveness
3. Psychophysiologic reactions	3. Truancy	3. School failure
	4. Running away from home	4. Delinquency
	5. Accident proneness	5. Psychosomatic symptoms
	6. Masochism	
	7. Self-destructive behavior	
	8. Boredom	
	9. Restlessness	
	10. Sexual acting-out	

From data of Glaser, K.: Ann. Prog. Child Psychiatry Child Dev. 1:345, 1968; Toolan, J. M.: Am. J. Orthopsychiatry 32:404, 1962; Cytryn, L., and McKnew, D. H.: Am. J. Psychiatry, 131:879, 1974.

masked symptoms of depression in children described by the three authors.

The difficulties in defining and conceptualizing depression in children are further complicated by studies of normal schoolchildren. Albert (1973) and Albert and Beck (1975) administered a short form of Beck's Depression Inventory to 63 children, 36 boys and 27 girls, between the ages of 11 and 15 years, enrolled in the 7th and 8th grades of a parochial school in suburban Philadelphia. The results were compared with scores obtained from depressed adults. According to the criteria set for adult depression, 33% of the children fell into the "moderate" to "severe depression" categories. It is unlikely, however, that one third of the children in this group were clinically depressed. The authors speculated that perhaps the inventory tapped some developmental problems which are characteristic of this age. Further analysis of the data indicated that over 50% of the children tested apparently had concerns about self-dislike, work difficulty, dissatisfaction and indecisiveness. Between 29 and 49% of the sample had thoughts and feelings of being a failure, fatigability, guilt, anorexia, social withdrawal, self-harm, pessimism and sadness.

CRITERIA FOR DIAGNOSING DEPRESSION IN CHILDREN

A subcommittee on clinical criteria for diagnosis of clinical depression in children, set up by the National Institute of Mental Health in 1975, recognized the following criteria as the essential clinical features of depression: (1) dysphoria and (2) generalized impairment of well-established habits, interests and sources of pleasure.

Associated features may include changes in self-esteem, guilt, personal and general pessimism or blaming others. It was stated that the depressive state must continue for a minimum of 4 weeks for the diagnosis of depression to be made. It was further emphasized that the diagnosis must be made on the basis of observation and information obtained from the parents as well as from other sources, such as teachers and other significant adults.

JUVENILE MANIC-DEPRESSION

Manic-depressive illness has traditionally been considered an adult disorder. Some investigators, however, hold that manic-depressive patients may display specific behavior in childhood which may be precursors of a cyclothymic personality or of adult manic-depression. Others state that some individuals may indeed manifest a juvenile version of the illness, which appears in childhood and which is characterized by rapid shifts in mood and behavior.

Formulation of diagnostic criteria and treatment plans for juvenile manic-depressive illness have been difficult and have received relatively little attention. Anthony and Scott (1960) offer the following suggestions for the diagnosis of juvenile manic-depression:

1. An abnormal psychiatric state at some time during the illness which approximates the classical description of manic-depression
2. A positive family history suggesting a predisposition to manic-depression
3. An early tendency toward a manic-depressive reaction as manifested by gradually increasing cyclothymic behavior and delirious manic or depressive outbursts during pyrexial illness
4. Two observed episodes of a recurrent or periodic illness with diagnostic agreement by different clinicians on the nature and identity of the episodes.
5. A diphasic illness showing swings of pathologic dimensions from states of elation to states of depression and vice versa
6. An endogenous illness, the phases of which show minimal reference to environmental events
7. A severe illness, as indicated by the need for hospitalization and sedation
8. An abnormal, underlying, extroverted personality, demonstrated by objective tests
9. Absence of features of schizophrenia or organic states

Redlich and Freedman (1966) condensed these criteria to 4 features:

1. There must be a distinct phasic disturbance of affect without intellectual and personality disintegration.

2. The episodes must be well defined. Neither very short periods of elation or depression nor lifelong depression or euphoria is characteristic.

3. Other manic-depressive or cyclothymic persons are present in the family.

4. Precipitating pathogenic factors are not conspicuous.

Feinstein and Wolpert (1973) reevaluated earlier criteria. They stated that rapidly shifting emotional states in children which do not seem related to environmental stress should be carefully evaluated as possible manifestations of manic-depressive illness. This is particularly important if the emotional states tend to remain prolonged and refractory to therapeutic intervention.

Various antidepressant drugs and lithium carbonate are being used in the treatment of juvenile manic-depression. Kelly et al. (1976) have reported on the long-term use of lithium in juvenile manic-depression and have found the drug to be very beneficial in reducing the frequency of these episodes.

Adolescent Depression

Adolescence normally includes frequent crises and upheavals. Brief episodes of depression are quite common. A brief review of the normal psychological development of adolescents is provided in the following paragraphs in order to better understand the episodic depression that can occur during this phase of development.

Anna Freud (1958) regards most adolescent reactions as prototypes of developmental disturbances. According to her, the primary cause of emotional problems in adolescents is the emergence of sexual and aggressive drives as a result of physical and endocrinologic changes. The adolescent runs the risk of having his new genital urges attach themselves to his old love objects (parents and siblings). To ward off these incestual fantasies, the adolescent completely discards the previous love objects by displaying indifference toward them or by openly revolting against their beliefs and conventions. Erikson (1956), although subscribing to a similar formulation, assigns sociological factors a much greater role in the genesis of adolescent problems. Osterrieth (1969), following Piaget's ideas on intellectual development, considers the adolescent's opposition to the values of the adult world an exercise of his newly developed powers of abstract thinking, which necessarily involve philosophic doubts and debates before the acceptance of adult life patterns.

All adolescents need to establish an identity of their own—some kind of personal answer to the age-old question, "Who am I?" Adolescents clearly are not all alike and do not all face the same environmental demands.

Problems confronting a socioeconomically deprived youth from a broken home living in a segregated urban ghetto are vastly different from the problems faced by an economically favored adolescent from a loving and protective suburban family.

Becoming psychologically independent of his parents is not a simple matter for an adolescent. He is likely to be ambivalent about independence. He may desire to be a free agent, but he may just as truly want the security and lack of responsibility that are associated with continuing dependence. As a result, he may suffer personal conflict over his independence needs. The ease with which this conflict is resolved in the direction of greater independence usually depends to a large extent on past and present relationships with his parents. The parents who encourage increasing autonomy as the child grows older but who still retain an interest in and some responsibility for the adolescent's decisions are likely to promote both responsibility and independence. Autocratic or authoritarian parents, on the other hand, tend to stifle the orderly acquisition of independent behavior, while indifferent or completely permissive parents may fail to encourage the development of responsibility.

Although most adolescents sooner or later confront the need to earn a living and to make their own way as independent members of society, there are some who fall by the wayside and become alienated from society.

Alienation from society is expressed in various ways:

1. Developmental estrangements. Keniston (1965) described a group of youths who felt that they had somehow lost touch with their real selves and who felt that much of what they did was empty, flat and devoid of meaning.

2. Student activism. Some youths extend their struggle for independence from their family to the rest of the society. They become actively involved in changing society through political protests. The student protests of the 1960s are illustrative of such activism.

3. Cultural alienation. In contrast to the politically involved or socially concerned protester, the culturally alienated youth is far too pessimistic and too firmly opposed to the system to wish to demonstrate his disapproval in any public way. His demonstrations of dissent are private—nonconforming behavior, ideology and dress, personal experimentation with deviant behavior and, above all, efforts to intensify his own subjective experience. He shows distaste for and lack of interest in politics and society.

4. Dropping out. While culturally alienated youth may be said to have dropped out spiritually and intellectually from middle-class culture, they have not found a substitute for it. Nihilistic and pervasively pessimistic, such youth remain in but not of the familiar middle- and upper-class cul-

ture. In contrast, the social dropout physically abandons his middle-class surroundings and lives a life outside the formal structures and roles of society, e.g., hippies.

Mood swings are often regarded as an inherent part of adolescence. The adolescent may appear uninterested in anything one moment, then preoccupied with trivia the next. He loses interest quickly, even in his most prized activities, then frantically seeks ways to entertain himself. Depression is expressed by withdrawal, regressive activities, aggressive activity, agitation and hypersexuality. He may alternate between overwhelming fatigue and inexhaustible energy. The fatigue is out of proportion to daily activity. He may also complain of excessive tiredness upon awaking in the morning in spite of an adequate amount of sleep.

Many depressed youngsters complain of difficulty in concentration, which may lead to problems with schoolwork and achievement. Grades may suddenly drop from A to C, to the amazement of teachers and parents. A depressed adolescent may engage in various delinquent activities, such as abuse of drugs and alcohol, running away from home and stealing. These activities seem to serve the purpose of denying and warding off feelings of depression.

Some adolescents use sexual acting-out as a method of relieving their depression. They frantically seek to make meaningful contact with other youths through sexual intercourse. Quite often, as in the case of alcoholism, this activity produces further depression and guilt.

The primary cause of reactive depression in adults is a loss, which can be real or fantasized. Similar dynamics may apply in adolescents. Growing up is perceived by some adolescents as giving up the conflict-free and sheltered life of childhood. They may also become overwhelmed by society's demands to join the adult world, choose a vocation and work for a living. Some adolescents may also see the adult world as very disappointing, whereas previously they could not wait to join it. This disparity between expectation and reality may be interpreted as loss.

All adolescents suffer from some degree of depression. In fact, it may be considered a basic psychobiologic affective reaction which, like anxiety, becomes abnormal only when it persists for an undue length of time and when the adolescent is unable to make a developmentally appropriate adaptation to it.

Initially, most children react to loss with feelings of anger. In some youths, this is quickly followed by feelings of helplessness and resignation, leading to a state of apathy. The anger may be turned against oneself and may lead to acting-out behavior and self-punishment.

The manner of handling depression depends largely on what type of activities and peer groups are available to an adolescent. Most adolescents utilize socially sanctioned, though somewhat eccentric, ways of dealing with their depression. Others who are unable to utilize peer contact and activities fall by the wayside and become isolated and further depressed. Such an adolescent may resort to suicide in a stressful situation.

It is impossible to predict, however, which depressed adolescent is likely to attempt suicide. To understand his suicidal tendencies, a great deal of knowledge about the adolescent is necessary, derived from lengthy interviews and prolonged contact. One of the reasons for the difficulty in detecting early indicators of suicide is the adolescent's tendency to hide his true feelings from others.

Suicide

The total number of suicides in the United States is above 20,000 per year. It is frequently argued that this figure is 25–33% too low, as many suicides are labeled "accidents." The rate of suicide in the 15–24-year age group has been steadily rising and has almost caught up with the suicide rate of the adult population (Figure 7–1). In 1976, the suicide rate for the general population was about 12 per hundred thousand and for the 15–24-year age group was 10.5 per hundred thousand.

After accidents and homicide, suicide appears to be the most frequent cause of death among adolescents.

Suicide is nonexistent before the age of 5. It is rare between the ages of

Fig. 7-1. Suicide rates in children, adolescents and adults. From data of National Vital Statistics, U.S. Department of Health, Education, and Welfare.

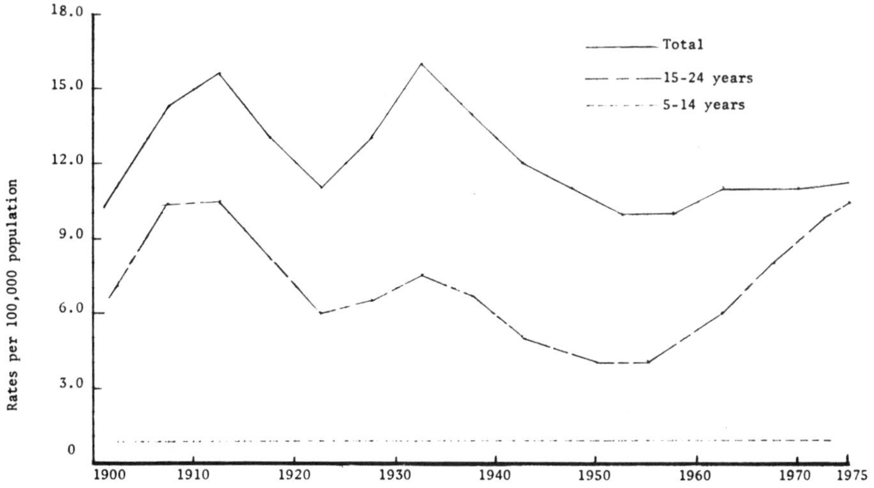

6 and 12. It is most common between 15 and 19 years of age. Several studies indicate that more girls than boys attempt suicide, but the probability of successful suicide is much greater for male attempters than for female attempters. Silverman (1968) found that girls attempted suicide 3–5 times more than boys, but the number of successful suicides was 3–4 times higher in boys than in girls. The ratio of attempted suicide to successful suicide is much higher in the adolescent population as a whole (as high as 120:1) than for the general population (approximately 8:1).

Suicide rates for nonwhites are lower than those for whites, with two important exceptions: (1) nonwhite females between the ages of 15–19 have a slightly higher rate than white females of the same age and (2) there has been a striking increase in suicide rate among nonwhite males of 15–24 years of age.

Precipitating Factors

There can be little doubt that the motivational factors underlying a suicidal attempt must be very strong in order to overcome the incredibly powerful survival instinct. Also, it seems impossible to characterize a suicide as "reasonable" without giving due consideration to associated psychiatric disturbances.

Most suicidal adolescents perceive the precipitating circumstances as unbearable and see suicide as a way of escaping them. The most common precipitating circumstances described by suicide attempters relate to family discord, breaking up of a love relationship, school problems and pregnancy. However, the circumstances mentioned immediately after a suicidal attempt often differ from what the youngster will say about it a few days later.

Some authors (Jacobziner, 1965) regard adolescent suicidal attempts as precipitous, impulsive reactions to stressful situations. However, Jacobs and Teicher (1967) seriously challenge the role of impulsiveness in adolescent suicidal behavior. In an intensive study of fifty 14–18 year olds, they concluded that adolescent suicide was not an impulsive act but rather the end result of a long history of relational problems, usually familial. Suicide attempts were the result of a complete breakdown of meaningful social relationships. Attempted suicide was the only perceived solution to this dilemma and came at the end of a long process. They divided this process into 3 stages:

1. A long history of parent-child relational problems (rejection, neglect, intense bitter quarrels, severe criticism)
2. An escalation period, beginning after the onset of adolescence, char-

acterized by intensification of older problems and more drastic attempts on the part of the adolescent at conflict resolution.

3. A final stage, involving a total breakdown in the parent-child relationship, leading to an attempted suicide to escape the stressful situation.

During the escalation period, adolescents become alienated from their families, and few meaningful ties are left with the family. Some of them embark on romantic involvements that appear as desperate attempts to secure love and security. Disappointments, frequently due to inflated expectations, lead to rupturing of love relationships and suicidal attempts.

The most common emotions associated with suicidal attempts are anger, aggression, feelings of helplessness and guilt. Aggression most often reflects feelings of spite toward one of the parents, the family or a friend, as well as a desire for revenge. The aggression, however, is turned against the self as punishment for having such emotions.

Suicidal attempts are also made to manipulate the environment and significant others and to gain attention. These motives, when discovered by family and friends, lead to further rejection of the adolescent and consequently to more serious suicidal attempts.

Toolan (1968) offered five underlying motives and reasons for suicidal attempts:

1. Anger at another person, internalized in the form of guilt and depression
2. A desire to gain affection and love or to punish others
3. Attempt to manipulate significant people in the environment
4. The desire to join dead relatives or friends
5. A reaction to psychotic hallucinations

Predisposing Factors

Teicher (1966) found that most of the suicidal adolescents in his group had a history of long-standing problems. Some of the significant features of their history are as follows:

1. Twenty percent of the adolescents had a parent who had attempted suicide.

2. Forty percent had a parent, relation or a close friend who had attempted suicide.

3. Seventy-two percent were from homes in which one or both of the natural parents were absent (divorced, separated or deceased).

4. Fifty percent belonged to low-income families.

5. Families showed marked residential mobility, an abnormal number of school changes and more siblings leaving home.

6. The adolescents had a long history of difficulties in academic achievement and in peer relationships.

7. In summary, this study suggests that suicidal adolescents are much more subject to unexpected separations from meaningful social relationships.

These findings seem to be fairly typical of many other studies. The majority of suicidal adolescents seem to have a great deal of difficulty with their parents throughout their childhood. They also seem less capable of adapting to their rejecting and chaotic environment. Among the more significant factors prevalent in the histories of these youngsters are the following types of disturbed family relationships: passive, inefficient father, domineering, cold, rejecting mother, absent father or mother (due to death, separation or divorce), severe marital problems between the parents, sexual molestation of girls by father and bitter quarrels between the parents and children.

In addition to a very frequent history of early losses, early rejection appears quite common. Early rejection by the parents creates a bad self-image in the child. Awareness of parental rejection becomes very acute during adolescence, when self-examination and identification are quite intense. In general, the initial reaction is anger. The rejecting parents have convinced the child over the years that he is "no good," "a black sheep of the family" or a "rotten apple." These self-labels arouse a feeling of worthlessness and apathy. The initial anger is turned inward and is transformed into guilt and depression.

Another important predisposing factor appears to be an excessively dependent relationship between the adolescent and his parents. In fact, the extreme dependency appears to have existed throughout childhood. Societal demands to become independent make the adolescent very anxious. Also reawakening of the Oedipus complex during adolescence often causes guilt feelings and consequent self-destructive tendencies. The intensity of the Oedipus complex is much greater with excessive dependency. These adolescents have low self-esteem, excessive intense guilt and severe superego. They are highly self-critical. Their self-hate appears to be related to the fact that they are unable to break the primary ties with their parents.

The various predisposing factors may be summarized as follows:

1. Long-standing relationship problems since childhood
2. Escalation of relationship problems—beyond levels and intensities normally characteristic of adolescence
3. Progressive failure of previously successful adaptive techniques
4. Chain reaction leading to further isolation and hopelessness
5. Mental process of justifying suicide

Suicidal Behavior

Several studies (Silverman, 1968) have investigated the questions of when, where and how the suicide is attempted. Ingestion of chemicals (primarily drugs) is the most popular method of attempted suicide. The means of suicide are, however, related to the age and the purpose of the attempter. Table 7–2 presents data on more violent methods of attempted suicide, such as running in front of a car or throwing oneself in front of a subway train. There appears to be a relationship, at least in the majority of cases, between the means of suicide and the degree of intent to succeed. It is less common for a violent attempt to fail, while ingestion of drugs is frequently detected before the suicide is successful.

There seems to be a logical tie between place of suicidal attempt and motivation. The suicidal attempt is likely to have more impact if it is committed or attempted in close proximity to the person or persons who are seen as being contributory to or the cause of the attempt.

Suicides are more frequent in the spring than in any other season, with the months of March, April and May having the highest averages. The months with the lowest number of suicides are the winter months of November, December and January.

Suicidal Adolescents

Most suicidal adolescents are of average intelligence. Reese (1967) found that in a group of 164 adolescents who attempted suicide (80% were female), 50% were doing D and F academic work at the time of the attempt, and 33% were doing A or B work. Fifty-nine percent had an I.Q. of 120 or more, and 23% had an I.Q. of 90 or below. Reese believes that

TABLE 7–2.—METHODS OF SUICIDE ATTEMPTS

	SEX		TOTAL	
METHOD OF SUICIDE ATTEMPT	MALE	FEMALE	NO.	%
Narcotic drugs	269	1,232	1,501	86.9
Hanging and strangulation	24	17	41	13.1
Shooting	4	1	5	
Gas poisoning	14	18	32	
Leaping from heights	8	10	18	
Throwing self before vehicle	1	6	7	
Drowning	5	13	18	
Cutting self	15	51	66	
Swallowing sharp objects	6	1	7	
Other methods	5	27	32	

From data of Jacobziner, H.: J.A.M.A. 191:7, 1965.

doing poorly in school precipitates the "mental condition" out of which suicidal tendencies germinate and also notes that the subjects were most often isolates who did not partake in extracurricular activities. They were the individuals whom no one seemed to know. Thus, doing poorly in school coupled with social introversion may be an important social indicator and precursor of suicidal tendencies.

There are various patterns of maladaptive behavior which are evident in suicidal adolescents. Otto (1964) described various personality disorders found in a large group of suicidal adolescents, of which the most common was a hysterical and immature personality.

Although personality disorders and depression are the most common psychiatric diagnoses associated with suicidal adolescents, schizophrenia is not a rare occurrence. Haider (1968) found only 2 schizophrenics in 64 cases of suicidal adolescents. Winn and Halla's sample, however, had an overabundance of schizophrenic adolescents—70% of the 70 adolescents were diagnosed as schizophrenic (1966). In the same study, another 15% were described as psychotics with organic brain damage. About 55% of all the subjects reported having received auditory hallucinatory instructions to kill themselves. Being from an institution, this study, however, had a very biased population. In a general population of suicidal adolescents, the occurrence of schizophrenia is estimated to be between 2 and 5%.

Presuicidal Behavior

Much thought has been given to the possibility of prescreening for suicide. Attempts have been made to determine the characteristics of persons on the verge of committing suicide. Otto (1964) studied, retrospectively, behavioral changes during the 3 months preceding the suicidal attempts of 581 Swedish adolescents under the age of 21 years. The behavioral changes studied were divided into five categories.

1. Conspicuous changes in social behavior, such as problems at work, in school, in personal hygiene and excessive drinking
2. Personality changes of an extroverted nature, such as increased irritability, aggressiveness, peevishness and unstable, fluctuating mood
3. Neurotic symptoms, such as anxiety, anguish, sleep disturbances, headache and tics
4. Depressive symptoms
5. Psychotic symptoms, such as delusions of influence and persecution and hallucinations of voices commanding suicide.

Although most adolescents had symptoms falling within more than one category, the largest group (38%) expressed primarily depressive symptoms, the next largest group showed symptoms of a neurotic character

(30%), while psychotic symptoms (3.2%) constituted the smallest group.

Otto concluded that the symptoms most characteristic of future suicides during the months preceding the suicidal attempt are depression and neurotic symptoms, such as anguish, unrest, sleep difficulties and psychosomatic symptoms. The extroverted symptoms of increased aggressiveness, increased irritability, labile mood and social behavior disturbances are unusual. In schizophrenic youth, one finds a flaring up of purely psychotic symptoms.

Sneidman (1968) classified all intimations and hints of and clues to suicide into four broad types:

1. Verbal hints—these may be expressed directly or indirectly. An example of a direct verbal hint would be such statements as "I am going to end it all," or "If such and such happens, I'll kill myself." Indirect verbal hints are more subtle and may be expressed by such statements as "You won't have to put up with me much longer."

2. Behavioral hints—which may also be expressed directly or indirectly. A direct behavioral hint would be a threat of suicide or an actual suicide attempt. An indirect behavioral hint often consists of preparatory actions, such as taking a lengthy trip to meet old relatives or putting affairs in order.

3. Situational clues—these clues are frequently expressed in stressful situations. For example, financial difficulties, family discord or friendship problems may drive some persons to excessive anxiety, frustration and, eventually, a suicidal attempt. Knowledge of a person's past history and his reaction to different life situations may provide clues to his probable response to new situations.

4. Syndromatic clues—these clues consist of the concomitant appearance of certain symptoms, such as depression, disorientation and defiance. Disoriented people are apt to be delusional and hallucinatory and are in great danger, as they may respond to hallucinations in such a way as to endanger their lives. A willful and defiant person dying of cancer may kill himself by jumping out the window rather than passively submitting to the disease.

Singer and Blumenthal (1969) have investigated suicidal clues in hospitalized psychotic patients, a group very reluctant and unlikely to express their suicidal ideation openly. They have identified 14 clues which indicate suicidal intent on the part of psychotic as well as nonpsychotic patients:

1. Dire predictions and morbid dreams
2. Verbalizations of aggression and revenge which may be directed toward the patient's own family and friends
3. Strong feelings of self-recrimination, or self-accusation in hallucinations

4. Expressions of despair and hopelessness about the inability to recover or leave the hospital
5. Loss of life force and profound resignation and indifference to death
6. Clinical symptoms, such as anorexia, insomnia or impotence, masking a more serious depressive state
7. Doubts regarding the worth of life and of living
8. Loss of a loved person in reality or fantasy
9. Loss of emotion in sexual fantasies
10. Psychosomatic delusions with morbid content, such as having an incurable disease
11. Emergence of a smiling depression—after a person makes up his mind to kill himself, he may become overtly cheerful and active
12. Breakthrough of latent homosexual tendencies, especially when a man is in close proximity with other men.
13. Significant statements in correspondence—letters written to friends may indicate suicidal intentions
14. Changes in attitude toward personal possessions—patients who refuse to spend their money on new clothes or other necessary items often do not intend to be around to use or enjoy such items.

Estimating the Seriousness of a Suicidal Intent

Many adolescents come to medical attention only after making a suicidal attempt. In such instances, one of the major tasks is to evaluate the seriousness of the suicidal intent and the likelihood of a repetition of the suicidal attempt.

An initial distinction should be made on the basis of whether mental examination reveals the adolescent to be psychotic or nonpsychotic.

Suicidal attempts associated with an acute psychotic condition are frequently related to the nature of the delusions and the hallucinations. This combination is extremely serious, as the attempter is likely to follow the commands of the "voices" or "visions" directing him to endanger or take his life. Two illustrative cases:

1. A 14-year-old girl was hospitalized after she injured her face and arms while trying to jump out of a third-floor apartment window. Her grandmother had died a few weeks earlier, and the girl had been very close to the grandmother. At the time of admission to the hospital, she reported that her grandmother was in the room and was asking her to join her. Her attempt to jump out the window had been in response to this hallucination.

2. A 15-year-old girl was hospitalized because she was trying to get away from "awful creatures" that were crowding her room. She had been caught in the act of jumping out a window. The visual hallucinations occurred after a bad LSD trip.

Most suicidal adolescents, however, are not psychotic, and it is much more difficult to determine the seriousness of their intent. Some estimate of the seriousness of suicide attempts on the part of nonpsychotic youths can be made on the basis of certain factors, such as age, sex, racial background, previous suicidal attempts, peer relationships and method of attempt. The importance of each of these factors has been investigated by several studies.

In a follow-up study of 38 hospitalized suicidal adolescents, Stanley and Barter (1970) found that about half of them continued self-destructive behavior after discharge. Those who attempted suicide after discharge were found to have less adequate peer relationships, were less likely to be living with their parents and had more social agency contact than those who did not make further suicidal attempts.

Similarly, Barter et al. (1968) followed 45 discharged youths who had been hospitalized for suicidal attempts and assessed them on 5 variables: living situation, parental loss, social life, social agency contact and school adjustment. They found that a majority (58%) of those making additional suicidal attempts after hospitalization did not live with their families. Either they were living alone, were in a psychiatric hospital or were in a foster home. In comparison, 84% of those not making suicidal attempts after discharge were living with their families. Of the adolescents making repeat suicidal attempts, 68% reported minimal or no social life, while 88% of those making no additional suicidal attempts reported an active social life. An active social life was defined as a minimum of one date per week or some sort of organized group activity, such as skating, team sports or social club meetings. Repeat attempters had greater contact with social agencies, such as a welfare agency, a mental health clinic or a mental hospital. Most of the 45 suicidal adolescents had done poorly in school.

Information with regard to the intent and planning of a suicidal attempt is very important but is frequently difficult to obtain. Generally, the more a youngster has considered and selected a particular time, place and method for his act (by which he maximizes both lethality and isolation from potential rescuers), the greater is the probability that he will kill himself. The intent is generally less serious if a suicidal attempt is made in order to manipulate other persons or the environment. The presence of severe guilt, depression and feelings of helplessness and hopelessness make suicidal intent more serious.

Most suicidal attempts appear to be impulsive, resulting from a temporary emotional upset and not a desire to die. They may, however, end fatally due to miscalculation and/or delay in obtaining prompt and appropriate treatment. Every suicidal attempt should be taken seriously and should be carefully evaluated. It should be kept in mind that at least 25% of all suicidal attempts are repeat attempts.

Tuckman and Youngman (1968) developed a scale for identifying persons likely to repeat a suicidal attempt (Table 7–3) on the basis of studying 1,112 adults who had attempted suicide. Most of these items are also applicable to adolescents. A total score of 14 is possible on the scale (simply adding up the factors falling in the high-risk category), but the actual scores ranged from 0 to 10, with a median of 2.6. With a score of 4 or more, repeat suicide rate was quite high, 35.2 per thousand. The authors concluded that there are factors, personal and social, that are associated with higher risk and that risk-related factors can be combined into a quantitative

TABLE 7–3.—RISK-RELATED FACTORS AMONG ATTEMPTED SUICIDES

FACTORS	HIGH-RISK CATEGORY	LOW-RISK CATEGORY
Age	Between 15–19 years	Under 15 years
Sex	Male	Female
Race	White	Nonwhite
Marital status	Separated, divorced, widowed	Single, married
Employment or educational status	Unemployed, out of school	Employed, in school
Living arrangement	Alone	With others
Health	Poor (acute or chronic) condition in the 6-month period preceding the attempt	Good
Mental condition	Nervous or mental disorder, mood or behavioral symptoms, including alcoholism	Presumably normal, including brief situational reactions
Method	Hanging, firearm, jumping, drowning	Use of cutting or piercing objects, gas or CO, poison, combination of methods
Potential consequences of method	Likely to be fatal	Harmless, illness producing
Police description of suicide's condition	Unconscious or semiconscious	Presumably normal, disturbed, drinking, physically ill, other
Suicide note	Yes	No
Previous attempt or threat	Yes	No
Disposition	Admitted to psychiatric evaluation center	Discharged to self, relative; referred to family doctor, clergyman, or social agency, or other

From Tuckman, J., and Youngman, W.: In Resnick, H. L. (ed.): *Suicidal Behaviors: Diagnosis and Management* (Boston: Little, Brown and Co., 1968). Used by permission.

scale for identifying high-risk and low-risk groups among attempted suicides.

Children Who Threaten to Kill Themselves

There are large numbers of children who have not attempted suicide but who have threatened to kill themselves during various frustrating situations. It is important to evaluate the seriousness of their intent. Winn and Halla (1966) studied 70 children under 15 years of age who had threatened to kill themselves. They were hospitalized for various associated emotional problems. In this group of 70 children, 40 were boys and 30 were girls. There were 25 boys below 10 years of age, 10 boys between 10 and 12 years of age, and 5 boys between 12 and 15 years of age. In contrast, there were 5 girls below 10 years of age, 10 girls between 10 and 12 years of age, and 15 girls between 12 and 15 years of age. Fifty-seven percent of the boys had threatened to jump from a height, 33% had threatened to cut or stab themselves, 15% had threatened to run in front of a car or train, 12% had threatened to choke or hang themselves and 10% had threatened to take poison. Among the girls, 47% had threatened to jump from a height, 20% to run in front of a car or train and 17% to choke or hang themselves. The percentages add up to more than 100% because many of the children had threatened suicide by more than 1 means. Thirty percent of these children had actually carried out their initial threats by jumping out of a low window, swallowing pills or cutting themselves. Fifty percent of the children had the means at their immediate disposal, in that they were at an open window, had pills or held a knife, but went no further. Twenty percent of the children did no more than verbalize an intention to kill themselves. The degree to which the threat was carried out bore no relationship to the degree of emotional disturbance.

Common Misconceptions about Suicide

Pokorny (1968) feels that there are a surprisingly large number of people in the general population who harbor false information about suicidal attempts by adolescents. Some of these misconceptions are presented in Table 7–4.

Management of Suicidal Children

All suicidal attempts should be taken seriously. Although suicidal attempts may vary in severity and intent, even the least serious gesture is intended to communicate something important about the person's life.

TABLE 7–4.—FACTS AND MISCONCEPTIONS ABOUT SUICIDAL BEHAVIOR

MISCONCEPTIONS	FACTS
People who talk about suicide will not commit it	60–80% of all suicides have communicated their intent
Suicide happens without warning	Often a direct statement of suicidal intent is made
Suicide and attempted suicide are behaviorally in the same class	They are qualitatively and motivationally very different
Suicide involves only a specific class of people	Suicide seems to depend more on the degree of integration of the individual with his culture
"Good circumstances" generally preclude suicide	Many professionals as well as youths from well-to-do families commit suicide
In the United States, more Protestants than Catholics commit suicide	There is some sketchy evidence from Europe for this, but it is not unequivocally correct
Motives or causes of suicide are readily established	There is often multiple and complexly interwoven causality
All suicidals are depressives	Neurotics, schizophrenics and passive-aggressives are also candidates
A terminally ill patient is an unlikely suicide	Many terminally ill people commit suicide
It is a "crazy," "insane" act	It is often attempted by normal people for rational, logical reasons

From data of Pokorny, A.D.: In Resnick, H. L. (ed.): *Suicidal Behaviors: Diagnosis and Management* (Boston: Little, Brown and Co., 1968). Used by permission.

One of the most important initial observations that the physician must make about the suicidal youth is whether delusions or hallucinations are present. Although acute psychosis associated with suicidal attempt is rare, it nevertheless does occur. Management of such children requires an extreme degree of caution. They should be protected by using whatever physical and chemical restraints are necessary. Such children require immediate hospitalization and should be restricted to one room, especially designed to foil attempts to jump out of the window. There should be an adult (nursing personnel, a parent or a relative) present in the child's room at all times until the intensity of the delusion and hallucination has subsided to the point where the patient is no longer responding to them. The major tranquilizers (e.g., phenothiazines) are of great assistance in the management of the initial acute phase. Tranquilizers are prescribed in moderate to high doses, depending upon the response of the child. They may later be combined with antidepressants, such as Elavil, depending upon the degree of manifest depression.

Should a nonpsychotic adolescent who has just made a first suicidal attempt be sent home or admitted to the hospital?

The seriousness of the suicidal attempt should first be assessed on the basis of the factors discussed in the previous sections before arriving at such a decision. Efforts should be made to determine the underlying motivation and intent of the attempter. A youngster may be sent home if the family is intact and concerned, peer contact and social relationships appear adequate, academic achievement is average, suicidal intent appears to be the manipulation of the environment and the act was impulsive rather than well planned. In cases of doubt, especially when the youngster is withdrawn and does not communicate, hospitalization is the treatment of choice. The purpose of such hospitalization is the observation of the child and the planning of further treatment.

Suicidal acts are the result of a complete breakdown of meaningful communication and social relationships and may represent a desperate attempt at changing an unbearable environmental situation. Every suicidal attempt is a cry for help and should be taken seriously. Every youth who has threatened or attempted suicide must be handled with a definite plan of treatment.

If the suicidal attempt was intended to escape an intolerable environment, an immediate goal of therapy may be to modify the environment of the child enough to make it tolerable to him. This goal may be best accomplished using some type of crisis intervention and family therapy. The family therapy should be aimed at understanding and then modifying communication patterns in the family system. Both parents, all siblings, grandparents and significant others may be included in the family therapy. The family therapy approach to the suicidal patient emphasizes that the suicidal attempt is a product of factors and forces in the family system. Marital relationships, the relationships between the parents and the siblings, as well as the relationships among the siblings, are explored, and the problems in these relationships are highlighted.

Individual therapy for the suicidal adolescent is rarely the treatment of choice, at least in the beginning. Most of these adolescents are very quiet, do not communicate their feelings well and are uncomfortable in individual therapy sessions. After a period of family therapy, however, the adolescent may feel comfortable enough to engage in individual therapy.

REFERENCES

Albert, N.: Evidence of Depression in an Early Adolescent School Population. Unpublished manuscript, Villanova, Pa., 1973.

Albert, N., and Beck, A. T.: Incidence of depression in early adolescence: A preliminary study, J. Youth Adolescence 4:301, 1975.

Anthony, J., and Scott, P.: Manic-depressive psychosis in childhood, J. Child Psychol. Psychiatry 1:53, 1960.
Barter, J. T., Swahack, D. O., and Todd, D.: Adolescent suicidal attempts: a follow-up study of hospitalized patients, Arch. Gen. Psychiatry 19:523, 1968.
Connell, H. M.: Depression in childhood, Child Psychiatry Hum. Dev. 4:71, 1972.
Cytryn, L., and McKnew, D. H.: Factors influencing the changing clinical expression of the depressive process in children, Am. J. Psychiatry 131:879, 1974.
Erikson, E.: The problem of ego identity, J. Am. Psychoanal. Assoc. 4:56, 1956.
Feighner, J. P., Robins, E., Guze, S. B., et al.: Diagnostic criteria for use in psychiatric research, Arch. Gen. Psychiatry 26:57, 1972.
Feinstein, S. C., and Wolpert, E. A.: Juvenile manic-depressive illness, J. Am. Acad. Child Psychiatry 12:123, 1973.
Freud, A.: Adolescence, *Psychoanal. Study Child* 13:255, 1958.
Glaser, K.: Masked depression in children and adolescents, Ann. Prog. Child Psychiatry Child Dev. 1:345, 1968.
Haider, I.: Suicidal attempts in children and adolescents, Br. J. Psychiatry 114:1133, 1968.
Jacobs, J., and Teicher, J. D.: Broken homes and social isolation in attempted suicides of adolescents, Int. J. Soc. Psychiatry 13:139, 1967.
Jacobziner, H.: Attempted suicide in adolescents, J.A.M.A. 191:7, 1965.
Kallman, F. J.: *Heredity in Health and Mental Disorders* (New York: W. W. Norton, 1953).
Kelly, J. T., Koch, M., and Buegel, D.: Lithium carbonate in juvenile manic-depressive illness, Dis. Nerv. Syst. 37:90, 1976.
Keniston, K.: *The Uncommitted* (New York: Harcourt, Brace and World, 1965).
Lewis, C.: *A Grief Observed* (New York: The Seabury Press, 1961).
McConville, B. J., Boag, L. C., and Purohit, A. P.: Three types of childhood depression, Can. Psychiatr. Assoc.'J. 18:133, 1973.
Osterrieth, P. A.: Adolescence: Some Psychological Aspects, in Caplan, G., and Lebovici, S. (eds.): *Adolescence* (New York: Basic Books, Inc., 1969).
Otto, U.: Changes in behavior of children and adolescents preceding suicidal attempts, Acta Psychiatr. Scand. 40:386, 1964.
Parker, C.: Seeing and finding a lost object: evidence from recent studies of the reaction to bereavement. II, Soc.'Sci. Med. 4:187, 1970.
Pokorny, A.: Myths about Suicide, in Resnik, H. L. (ed.): *Suicidal Behavior: Diagnosis and Management* (Boston: Little, Brown and Co., 1968, pp. 57-72).
Redlich, F., and Freedman, D. X.: *The Theory and Practice of Psychiatry* (New York: Basic Books, 1966).
Reese, F.: School-age suicide: The educational parameters, Diss. Abstr. 27:2895, 1967.
Renshaw, D. C.: Suicide and depression in children, J. Sch. Health 44:487, 1974.
Report of the Subcommittee on Clinical Criteria for Diagnosis of Depression in Children, in Schulterbrandt, J. G., and Raskin, A. (eds.): *Depression in Childhood: Diagnosis, Treatment, and Conceptual Models* (Washington, D.C.: U.S. Govt. Printing Office, 1977).

Silverman, C.: *The Epidemiology of Depression* (Baltimore, Johns Hopkins University Press, 1968, pp. 157–202).
Singer, R., and Blumenthal, I.: Suicide clues in psychotic patients, Ment. Hyg. 53:346, 1969.
Sneidman, E.: Preventing suicide, Bull. Suicidology 4:19, 1968.
Stanley, E., and Barter, J.: Adolescent suicidal behavior, Am. J. Orthopsychiatry 40:87, 1970.
Teicher, J. D.: Treatment of the Suicidal Adolescent—the Life-line Approach. Excerpta Medica, Itnernational Congress Series No. 15. Proceedings of the World Congress of Psychiatry (Amsterdam: Excerpta Medica Foundation, 1967, p. 747).
Teicher, J. D., and Jacobs, J.: Adolescents who attempt suicide: Preliminary findings, Am. J. Psychiatry 122:1248, 1966.
Toolan, J. M.: Depression in children and adolescents, Am. J. Orthopsychiatry 32:404, 1962.
Toolan, J. M.: Suicide in Childhood and Adolescence, in Resnik, H. L. (ed.): *Suicidal Behavior: Diagnosis and Management* (Boston: Little, Brown and Co., 1968, pp. 220–227).
Tuckman, J., and Youngman, W.: Assessment of Suicide Risk in Attempted Suicides, in Resnik, H. L. (ed.): *Suicidal Behaviors: Diagnosis and Management* (Boston: Little, Brown and Co., 1968, pp. 190–197).
Weinberg, W. A., Rutman, J., Sullivan, L., et al.: Depression in children referred to an educational diagnostic center: Diagnosis and treatment, J. Pediatr. 83:1065, 1973.
Winn, D., and Halla, R.: Observation of children who threaten to kill themselves, Can.'Psychiatr. Assoc. J. 11:S283, 1966.

8/Childhood Psychoses

PSYCHOTIC ILLNESS in children was reported as early as the middle of the 18th century, but there was little serious scientific interest in this condition until a few decades ago. There have been a few studies of prevalence rates of early childhood psychosis (Lotter, 1966; Treffert, 1970), the figures reported for the United States and England ranging from 2/10,000 to 4.5/10,000.

Childhood psychosis is manifested as a group of conditions varying in clinical severity. Some of the clinical manifestations have been sufficiently clear-cut to warrant labeling as distinct disease entities, as is the case with autism, symbiotic psychosis and childhood schizophrenia. Very little is known about the etiology of these disorders.

Classification of psychosis in children is based primarily on differences in clinical severity and theoretical considerations regarding etiology. For purposes of this discussion and from the point of view of management, psychoses may be classified into 2 broad categories: acute and chronic. Each category is further subclassified on the basis of presumed etiology into organic and functional.

Acute Psychoses

Diagnostic Criteria

Although the etiology of an acute episode of psychosis may remain permanently obscure, the initial diagnosis is generally easy and is based upon the signs and symptoms of brain dysfunction: bizarre thinking, inappropriate expression of emotions, poor comprehension of reality, disturbance of level of consciousness and bizarre behavior.

While many organic diseases can cause episodes of acute psychosis, the following questions are helpful in differentiating between organic and nonorganic acute psychoses:

1. Is the symptom complex an acute psychiatric condition (functional psychosis), unrelated to any apparent organic disturbance?
2. Is the condition associated with primary organic involvement of the central nervous system?
3. Is it associated with acute, subacute or chronic disease with secondary involvement of the brain?

Differential diagnosis between acute functional psychosis and the acute psychosis caused by a known organic condition frequently presents a major challenge. A history of psychiatric disturbance strongly suggests a diagnosis of functional psychosis but does not rule out the possibility of an organic condition as the precipitating cause of the acute attack. Similarly, a positive history of past organic conditions does not exclude a functional psychotic episode precipitated by the stress and strains of the disease and an inability to cope with an unfavorable environment.

It is customary to distinguish between organic and functional psychoses on the basis of brain involvement: acute organic psychosis is suspected when the level of consciousness and the cognitive functions are moderately disturbed, with a positive diagnosis being made on the basis of the presence of an acute organic condition.

Organic conditions which give rise to acute psychotic episodes usually cause a diffuse cerebral dysfunction. Disturbances of consciousness and memory are of much greater intensity than those found in functional psychoses. The level of consciousness may deteriorate with the intensity of the organic condition, from fluctuating attention to inattention, somnolence and coma. Various cognitive and motor functions, such as memory, retention, recall, mathematical skills and ability to sustain a mental or motor task, are impaired.

Acute Functional Psychosis

Acute episodes of functional psychosis in young children are rare. Extreme withdrawal or severe agitation may be seen in very young children on separation from their parents. The commonly described functional childhood psychoses are of the insidious type and produce a deterioration in the child's behavior. There are sometimes acute episodes of excitement and bizarre behavior that occur concurrently with chronic conditions. These episodes may initially bring a child to the attention of a physician, but a careful history generally reveals the chronic nature of the problem.

Acute psychotic episodes are more frequent in early adolescence and midadolescence and resemble the psychoses of adult patients. Catatonic and paranoid types of schizophrenic reactions are commonly encountered as acute manifestations, while simple and hebephrenic types are inferred from a chronic progressive history of personality deterioration.

CATATONIC TYPE

Catatonia usually has an acute onset. It is characterized by phases of stupor and/or excitement. Frequently, a particular episode may manifest only one phase—either stupor or excitement. A stuporous catatonic adolescent presents as mute, with mask-like facies. The eyes may be closed but are frequently open and staring blankly downward. The patient may spend hours in one bodily position, such as lying in bed or standing immobile, seldom shifting his position. The condition is characterized by a high degree of negativism and automatism. The patient actively opposes all efforts to move him from the position he has assumed. The patient also refuses to dress or eat, although occasionally he may devour large amounts of food, especially when unobserved. Urine and feces may be retained for several days. Similarly, the patient may hold saliva in his mouth for a long time without swallowing. Some patients will carry out any verbal instructions, regardless of their absurd or even dangerous nature. The patient may show no reaction to feinting motions before the eyes, to pinpricks or to painful stimuli, and his stupor may be compared to a retreat into an intense, trance-like preoccupation. Although giving no indiciation whatsoever that he is at all aware of his surroundings, he may register the minute details of events occurring in his environment. On recovery, the patient may give a surprisingly full account of incidents occurring in his stupor. After a period of extremely variable duration, from a few days to several months, the patient may slowly, or at times suddenly, emerge from this profound regression. His interest, affect and behavior may become almost normal, or occasionally a patient may pass into a state of catatonic excitement.

Catatonic excitement is manifested as an unorganized and aggressive motor activity. It appears purposeless and stereotyped. There is little facial expression during the aggressive activity, which occurs without provocation in an impulsive and unpredictable manner. The patient may not sleep and eat for days. He may remain mute or talk incessantly.

The prognosis for catatonic schizophrenia is generally considered better than for other types. An adolescent may recover within a period of a few days or weeks. Repeated episodes, however, indicate a poor prognosis. The patient may recover only partially from a single episode and may deteriorate into other types of chronic schizophrenic reactions. Before the onset of an acute phase, there is usually a subacute phase, in which depression, discontent, inattention, preoccupation, withdrawal from social activities and uncommunicativeness with parents occur. This phase of disturbance is frequently interpreted as "teenage problems" and is ignored until the acute phase of stupor or excitement develops.

Paranoid Type

Paranoia is characterized by the presence of numerous delusions and hallucinations. Auditory hallucinations are the most common type. An adolescent may begin to hear voices which call him bad names or say derogatory things about him. Visual hallucinations are rare, and their presence alone may imply organic psychosis. Occasionally, preadolescent children may present with an acute onset of visual hallucinations which are quite elaborate in structure.

A 10-year-old girl was seen in the emergency room, where she appeared quite upset and frightened. Her mother reported that the girl was seeing a black goat with twisted, long horns who was about to attack her. She also occasionally saw a dog and a rabbit. These hallucinations appeared intermittently on an almost daily basis for four days. The girl was the 3rd of 5 siblings in an intact black family of a highly religious, Southern background. The mother had tried to help the daughter by suggesting she read the Bible whenever these hallucinations appeared. Reading the Bible seemed to dispel the hallucinations temporarily.

She was reported to be a fairly outgoing girl who related easily to peers and adults, did well in school and had no history of psychiatric illness in her family.

She was a fairly verbal child and responded well in intensive psychotherapy. Phenothiazines were administered. Hallucinations ceased within a period of four weeks after therapy. Phenothiazines were discontinued 4 months later, but psychotherapy was continued for a year. Precipitating causes seemed to be psychological and were related to her feelings of sexual attraction toward boys and fear of reprisal from her mother.

In younger children, it may be difficult at times to distinguish between a fantasy and a visual hallucination. An especially interesting form of imagery in childhood is the imaginary companion. This phenomenon is likely to occur some time between the ages of 3 and 10 years, usually earlier than later. The label "imaginary companion" is commonly applied to an imagined creature (person or animal) or thing that is unusually vivid. It is quite stable in characteristics (while it lasts), and it appears for varying lengths of time and then disappears in the sense that it loses its vividness, although it may remain as a memory. It is the unique product of a particular child's imagination. The companion usually occupies space and can be played with and talked to. Imaginary companions are far more real than the characters in a daydream. When a child talks to his imaginary companion, he is not like a person having hallucinations or hearing voices, for imaginary companions behave like companions, as opposed to most hallucinations, which intrude as overbearing figures or objects.

An imaginary companion serves various needs of the child, such as companionship, self-aggrandizement and release for forbidden impulses. It is a fairly benign condition and disappears when the parents pay attention to and support the child.

Acute Psychoses Caused By Known Organic Conditions

Acute infections, metabolic disorders, cardiovascular disturbances, drug ingestion and trauma may be associated with acute psychosis. In these conditions, psychotic symptoms result from a diffuse cerebral dysfunction.

INFECTION

Infection of the brain or other parts of the body may result in brain dysfunction, either by direct invasion of the brain or through toxic, hypoxic or allergic effects. Mild infections cause nonspecific changes, such as irritability, insomnia and restlessness. Severe infections may give rise to visual hallucinations, impairment of memory and alterations in consciousness.

CEREBROVASCULAR DISEASES

Cerebrovascular diseases include all morbid processes, primary or secondary, in which the blood vessels of the brain are involved. Although cerebrovascular accidents are frequently considered a clinical rarity in childhood, in actuality they are not infrequent and account for about 5% of admissions to a pediatric neurology service and 10% of pediatric pathology material. Children with congenital heart disease not uncommonly have cerebrovascular complications. Approximately 10% of patients with tetralogy of Fallot have cerebrovascular accidents, and 25% of all cardiac patients have evidence of cerebrovascular occlusion at autopsy. Blood dyscrasias add to these figures. Spontaneous cerebral hemorrhage secondary to a hematologic disorder is not uncommon and is found in 50% of leukemic children at necropsy. In the pediatric age group, arteriovenous malformations are ten times as common as intracranial aneurysm and are the most common cause of primary subarachnoid hemorrhage. Subarachnoid hemorrhage and subdural hematoma are especially likely to be associated with behavioral symptoms resembling acute psychosis.

EPILEPSY

Psychomotor seizures are frequently confused with acute psychotic symptoms. These seizures, which originate primarily in the temporal lobe of the brain, rarely occur in young children but are not uncommon in the preadolescent and adolescent years. These seizures usually occur without loss of consciousness but occasionally are associated with generalized grand mal seizures.

Perceptual distortions in psychomotor seizures may run the gamut from a mild sensory disturbance to a complex visual hallucination. Visual distortions may occur in the size of an object, as if it were receding or approaching. Objects may appear very small and distant or quite large. Similar distortions may occur in other sensory perceptions. Voices may be heard as if they were distant or very loud as if everyone was shouting. Olfactory hallucinations of a complex nature may occur.

Patients generally have a clear understanding and awareness of the nature of their perceptual distortions and recognize them as alien. Feelings of déjà vu (sudden feelings of intense familiarity) and jamais vu (feelings of unfamiliarity in a familiar situation) may also occur. A phenomenon of forced thought, in which a thought, word or sentence may intrude on consciousness, has also been described. This should be distinguished from obsessive thoughts, which are frequently associated with other obsessive-compulsive acts and anxiety.

Temporary emotional disturbances in the form of waves of fear, anxiety, despair, depression, pleasure, elation and serenity may also occur. Complex, stereotyped, automatic acts may be performed. These acts, which may be purposeful, are inappropriate to the situation.

The diagnosis of psychomotor seizure, in the absence of temporal lobe abnormality, lies at the borderline between psychiatry and neurology. A child with psychomotor seizure is more aware of the irrationality of his perceptual distortions than is a severely neurotic or a psychotic child. Most of these borderline cases require a thorough psychosocial evaluation to arrive at a definitive diagnosis.

TWILIGHT STATES

Twilight states associated with seizure disorders may also be confused with acute psychosis. A postictal twilight state may occur at the close of a grand mal seizure or perhaps after a period of sleep. The patient is usually awake but in a confused state, mumbling incoherently and fumbling with his clothing or other objects. These periods of confusion may last from minutes to (rarely) several days. Hallucinations and delusions may also be present. Such states usually terminate completely with surprising abruptness, generally with complete amnesia for these periods. An electroencephalogram recorded during this period reveals diffuse symmetrical slow activity, unlike the paroxysmal activity of the seizure state.

The ictal twilight state may be preceded by focal disturbances, usually of the temporal lobe. The patient may become disoriented and is only partially aware of his surroundings, and masticatory movements, lip-smacking, swallowing, fumbling with clothing and mumbling may occur. The period usually lasts from 5 to 10 minutes but may occasionally be prolonged.

HEAD TRAUMA

Injury to the head may be confined to the scalp or may involve fracture of the skull, concussion, contusion or laceration of the intracranial structures. It may be associated with bleeding in various compartments of meninges and brain. Signs and symptoms of acute head injury (especially extradural or subdural hematoma) may sometimes be confused with the acute onset of psychosis. This may occur in patients in whom a history of head injury is not available because of amnesia. Parents may bring a youngster to the emergency room because of acute agitation, confusion, delirium, perceptual distortions or extreme withdrawal. Existence of past behavioral and emotional problems may further obscure the diagnosis of head injury. Disturbances of orientation, memory and consciousness indicate an acute organic etiology.

BRAIN TUMORS

Patients with brain tumors rarely present with acute brain syndrome. Early diagnosis of cerebral tumor in children may be difficult and is frequently overlooked because of the child's unawareness of change, inability to express himself adequately or inability to understand and carry out some of the discriminating neurologic tests. Gradual changes in behavior and personality may suddenly merge into acute disturbances of behavior and perception and may, at times, be interpreted as acute psychosis.

LEAD INTOXICATION

Mental symptoms associated with lead poisoning may manifest as (1) acute delirious episodes and/or (2) progressive mental deterioration. Acute onset of symptoms is usually characterized by restlessness, confusion, outbursts of violent temper tantrums, visual hallucinations and delusions. Convulsions, when associated with mental symptoms, help clarify the diagnosis but represent a poor prognosis. These manifestations are frequently associated with physical symptoms of constipation, colic and vomiting.

Acute Alcoholic Psychosis

Numerous studies of younger populations, mostly in high schools, reveal that the use of alcohol has increased significantly in the 1970s. From 71 to 92% of American high-school students have tried alcohol at least once. Drinking beer at least once a week increases from 10% among 7th graders to 42% among 12th graders. At least 5% of all high-school students are considered problem drinkers. (Second Special Report to the U. S. Congress on Alcohol and Health, June 1974). With this continuous rise in alcohol consumption by adolescents, an increasing number of these youngsters are being seen in emergency rooms of general hospitals with signs of acute alcoholic intoxication.

Acute toxic reaction to alcohol may be manifested in the following forms: severe intoxication, blackouts, delirium tremens and alcoholic hallucinosis.

In severe intoxication, the adolescent is disoriented and confused and may suffer from illusions, transitory delusions and visual hallucinations. There is a great increase in activity level, impulsiveness and aggression, often to the point of destructiveness.

Occurrence of blackouts is fairly frequent. The adolescent may not recall his activities or behavior during the period just before or during the blackout.

Delirium tremens is associated with decrease in the blood level of alcohol. Its course usually runs 3 to 10 days, with recovery preceded by prolonged sleep, clearer consciousness and disappearance of hallucinations.

Acute alcoholic hallucinosis usually follows a prolonged drinking bout. Auditory hallucinations of a threatening nature are common. The patient is not confused, and the sensorium is fairly clear.

Metabolic Disorders

HYPOGLYCEMIA

Symptoms of hypoglycemia are quite variable and may at times be confused with acute psychosis or anxiety reaction. Symptoms of weakness, fainting, sweating, headache, hunger, muscle pains, sensory disturbances, confusion and hallucinations may occur. The ability to maintain normal serum glucose levels is frequently disturbed in infancy and childhood. This disturbance may result from multiple causes and may contribute to disorders of glycolysis, gluconeogenesis, absorption from the gastrointestinal tract and hyperinsulinism. Uncontrolled hypoglycemia may cause progressive cerebral damage resulting in epilepsy and mental retardation.

Most patients respond rapidly to restoration of a normal serum glucose level unless neurologic involvement is marked. Later, treatment should be designed to counteract the imbalance in glucose homeostasis.

PORPHYRIA

Hemoglobin (Hb) consists of protein (globin) and four heme groups. Heme consists of a porphyrin ring structure containing a chelated iron atom. Porphyrins are widely distributed in nature and are found both in plants and animals, where they serve vital metabolic processes.

Senescent red cells are removed from circulation by reticuloendothelial cells. Hb is liberated but is not reutilized as such. Amino acids released from the degradation of globin return to the general amino acid pool. The degradation of heme to bile pigment takes place in the reticuloendothelial cells. Heme is first transformed to biliverdin with the release of iron; the iron is then returned to the iron pool and is reutilized in the formation of Hb. Biliverdin is next reduced to bilirubin, which in turn is released from the reticuloendothelial cells into plasma, where it is bound to albumin and transported to the parenchymal cells of the liver. In the liver, it is conjugated with glucuronic acid and excreted into the bile. If the liver is unable to carry on this conjugation in the normal manner, there is a high indirect-acting bilirubin level in the blood. If there is obstruction of excretion of conjugated form via the biliary system, there is an increase in the direct-acting bilirubin in the blood.

Disease states that result from disordered porphyrin metabolism may be classified as follows:

- Disorders of porphyrin synthesis in erythrocytes
  - Porphyria (congenital) erythropoietica
  - Protoporphyria (congenital) erythropoietica
- Disorders of porphyrin synthesis in the liver
  - Porphyria hepatica
    - Intermittent acute
    - Hereditary coproporphyria
    - Cutanea tarda
    - Mixed type
- Acquired (toxic) porphyria

Intermittent acute porphyria is of the greatest interest to psychiatrists. It is a familial disorder, inherited as an autosomal dominant factor. It usually appears after puberty, though in rare cases it may occur in childhood. In this disorder, erythrocyte porphyrins are normal, but excessive quantities of zinc-complexed uroporphyrin I and III and coproporphyrin III are found in the urine. The porphyrin precursor, porphobilinogen, is found in the urine during an acute attack, and the finding of this monopyrrole is diagnostic.

The liver contains large quantities of porphyrin precursors and porphyrins, with recent evidence pointing to reduced activity of hepatic uroporphyrinogen synthetase as the fundamental defect.

Attacks of acute intermittent porphyria appear to be precipitated by factors that increase the activity of a liver enzyme (ALA synthetase), which is the rate-limiting enzyme in the synthesis of heme. Among the various factors reported to precipitate attacks of acute intermittent porphyria are pregnancy, endogenously derived 5, β-steroids, contraceptive pills, various sedatives (especially barbiturates), tranquilizers, anticonvulsants, sulfa drugs and methyldopa.

Clinical manifestations are varied. Abdominal colic (which can be of extreme severity), weakness, paresthesias of extremities, constipation, convulsions, coma, psychosis and hypertension may occur. Psychotic symptoms resemble those of acute brain syndrome.

Preventive measures include avoidance of alcohol, barbiturates or other liver toxins. Chloropromazine therapy is effective in relieving symptoms.

Nutritional Deficiencies

Nutritional deficiencies in children rarely cause psychotic symptoms. Primary manifestations are increased irritability, apathy and poor concentration. In severe cases, confusion and sensory disturbances in the form of hallucinations may occur.

Nutritional problems in adolescents have received increased attention in recent years. Poor eating and sleeping habits of adolescents may lead to nutritional deficiencies that cause poor concentration, obsessive ideas and, occasionally, delusion and hallucination.

NICOTINIC ACID DEFICIENCY (PELLAGRA)

Pellagra is characterized by a combination of symptoms involving the skin, digestive tract and central nervous system. Lesions are found on the dorsal parts of the skin of the hands. These lesions usually start as erythema, which progresses to darkly pigmented, rough, sharply demarcated and sunburn-like dermatosis. There is widespread gastrointestinal inflammation, with dysphagia, vomiting and attacks of diarrhea. Early mental symptoms include apathy, irritability and poor concentration. Later mental symptoms may include confusion, delusion and hallucinations.

Treatment consists of giving 10–25 mg of nicotinamide 3 times daily for 2 weeks, followed by adequate dietary preventative measures.

THIAMINE DEFICIENCY

Thiamine deficiency is rare. It causes fatty degeneration of the myocardium, edema of the heart and interstitial tissues. Myelin and axonal degeneration occur in the peripheral nerves. Physical symptoms include tachycardia, dyspnea, cyanosis, cardiomegaly, hepatomegaly, pulmonary edema, diarrhea, peripheral palsy and ataxia. The mental symptoms usually consist of apathy, irritability, poor concentration, sleep disturbances and confusion.

Systemic Lupus Erythematosus (SLE)

SLE is an immune complex disease, and its pathogenesis is related to deposition in the tissues of soluble immune complexes existing in the circulation. The trigger for the formation of immune complexes is not known, but data from animal studies suggest that the immune aberrations antedate the disease. Such drugs as the hydantoin compounds, procainamide and isoniazid can cause a syndrome related to systemic lupus erythematosus, which generally disappears when therapy is discontinued.

Females suffer from SLE more often than do males (8:1), with the typical onset being between the ages of 9 and 15 years. The manifestations of the disease depend on the organ involved with the immune complex deposition. Joint pains, myositis, weakness, fever, weight loss, skin lesions, hepatosplenomegaly, lymphadenopathy and renal involvement may all occur. Involvement of the central nervous system may produce focal neurologic signs as well as general behavior disorders, including psychosis, with acute delusions and hallucinations.

Treatment is primarily with steroids. There is general agreement that steroids should not be discontinued if psychiatric symptoms appear. Phenothiazine may be added for the treatment of psychotic symptoms.

Capgras Syndrome (Illusion of the Double)

The first systematized description of this syndrome was provided by the French psychiatrist Capgras. The salient features of this syndrome consist of the nonrecognition of a person or persons who are usually very close to the sufferer. The pivotal delusion centers around the idea that in the place of a well-known person, the patient is seeing an exceedingly clever fake, an imposter who is a carbon copy, as it were, of the original—a double. The sufferer believes that the imposter has perpetrated the ruse with the treacherous design of deceiving him. This syndrome was formerly considered a functional psychosis only. However, during the last decade a number of clinical studies have pointed to the possibility of an organic etiology, including an association with organic brain syndromes. Although the majority of reported cases are adults, a case of a waxing and waning Capgras phenomenon occurring as a sequel to postvaricella encephalitis in a 9-year-old boy was described by Nikolovski and Fernandez (1978).

Management of Acute Psychoses

Once a diagnosis of acute psychosis is made, the following considerations are helpful in the management of the patient:

1. Is there enough family support to treat the patient on a living at home basis?

2. Does the patient need protection from his suicidal or homicidal ideation?

3. Presence of a moderate to severe degree of confusion or delirium will require hospitalization.

4. Most patients with acute psychosis associated with an organic condition will require hospitalization for a complete investigaton of the suspected condition.

Patients without delirium, confusion and suicidal or homicidal ideation may be treated on an outpatient basis if the support of the family appears adequate.

Acute episodes of psychosis frequently require treatment with antipsychotic medications. Suspected organic conditions should always be explored first before using antipsychotic drugs. In emergency situations, however, acute episodes of excitement and aggression prompted by delusions or hallucinations may be treated with intramuscular administration of antipsychotic drugs. For example, Thorazine may be given in dosages of 0.25 to 0.5 mg/lb body weight by intramuscular injection. The maximum dosage of Thorazine for intramuscular injection for children up to 5 years of age is 40 mg/day; for 5–12 years of age, 75 mg/day. The injection should be given slowly, deep into the upper quadrant of the buttock. Because of the possible hypotensive effect, the patient should remain lying down for at least half an hour after the injection. After the initial excitement subsides, Thorazine should be given orally in maintenance doses (1 to 2 mg/lb body weight).

Acute functional psychoses requiring immediate treatment include patients with severe delusions and/or hallucinations causing excitement and aggression, catatonic patients and patients with suicidal intentions. Patients in a catatonic stupor require specialized intensive nursing care. These patients may have to be spoon-fed or tube-fed and helped with their bowel and bladder incontinence for weeks and sometimes for months. Antipsychotic drugs such as Stelazine, Taractan and Haldol are the drugs of choice and are given orally or intramuscularly.

A patient with delirium tremens (d.t.s) requires hospitalization and intensive nursing care. Administration of opiates and physical restraints should be avoided. Many of these patients have died struggling against bodily restraints or from the effects of deep sedation. Treatment should be directed at alleviating the agitation, correcting dehydration and nutritional deficiencies and treating and preventing the occurrence of epileptiform seizures.

The most commonly used drugs to alleviate agitation in d.t.s are chlordiazepoxide (Librium) and hydroxyzine (Atarax, Vistaril). Librium is given in 50–100 mg dosage intramuscularly or intravenously. This dose may be repeated every 2 to 4 hours as necessary. Alternatively, Vistaril is given,

50–100 mg intramuscularly, and may be repeated every 4 to 6 hours. Diazepam (Valium) 5–10 mg intramuscularly or intravenously is used initially to control recurrent seizures. This dose may be repeated every 2 to 4 hours as necessary. Occasionally, a paradoxical reaction of a hyperexcitation is reported with Valium. Diphenylhydantoin (Dilantin) 50–100 mg 3 times daily by mouth may be added for continued treatment to raise the threshold for seizure occurrence.

A dehydrated patient is treated with fluids fortified with vitamin B complex given orally or parenterally. Thiamine hydrochloride in daily doses of 200 mg may be given orally or intramuscularly.

Other forms of alcoholic intoxication, if not too profound, may be treated with 10–25 mg of Librium 4 times daily for 1 to 3 days without hospitalization. Severe intoxication, however, requires hospitalization and is treated with Librium or Atarax in the same dosages used in the treatment of d.t.s.

Patients with alcoholic hallucinosis may require hospitalization for withdrawal from alcohol. These patients frequently have underlying emotional problems and require continued treatment with antipsychotic drugs.

Chronic Psychoses

Diagnostic Criteria

Psychotic conditions seem to persist for the entire life of the individual, although variations in intensity and level of adjustment vary from time to time. Most psychotic children will adjust to the community's standard of acceptable social behavior with treatment. Childhood psychosis does not resemble the fully developed clinical picture seen in psychotic adults. The most frequent manifestation of psychosis in children is a disturbed relationship of the affected child with adults and other children. Such a child is seclusive, withdrawn and a daydreamer who takes little part in activities involving other children. It is generally quite difficult for the physician to elicit and detect disturbances of thought during the first contact, since it takes a great deal of time for such a child to relate to other adults. The reports of parents or other observers may be relied upon to suggest the presence of thought disorder. Most frequently, thought disorder in a severely psychotic child is reflected in his bizarre and inappropriate behavior and in diminished expression of emotions. A history of bizarre behavior is usually cited by the parents and may consist of rigid, stereotyped and immature behavior, while inappropriate emotions may be expressed in the form of unwarranted explosiveness and unprovoked anger.

Since the manifestations of chronic psychoses vary among different patients as well as in the same individual at different times, diagnostic criteria for these conditions have varied over the years and remain somewhat controversial. Potter (1933) used the following criteria: (1) generalized retraction of interest from the environment, (2) deviant thinking, feeling and acting, (3) disturbances of thought, manifested by blocking, symbolism, condensation, perseveration, incoherence and diminution of speech, sometimes to the extent of mutism, (4) defect in emotional rapport, (5) diminution, rigidity and distortion of affect, (6) alterations of behavior, involving increased motility, decreased motility (including complete immobility) or bizarre behavior with a tendency to perseveration or stereotyping.

Bender (1956) considered schizophrenic children to be developmentally retarded and neurologically damaged. She felt that schizophrenic children revealed pathology in every area of behavior and cognition associated with the functioning of the central nervous system, be this vegetative, motor, perceptive, intellectual, emotional or social.

The British Working Party under Mildred Creak's chairmanship published (1961) a set of nine points by which a diagnosis of schizophrenic syndrome might be made: (1) gross and sustained impairment of emotional relationships with people, (2) apparent unawareness of one's own personal identity to a degree inappropriate to one's age, (3) pathologic preoccupation with particular objects or certain characteristics without regard to their accepted functions, (4) sustained resistance to change in the environment, combined with striving to maintain or restore sameness, (5) abnormal perceptual experience (in the absence of discernible organic abnormality), implied by excessive, diminished or unpredictable responses to sensory stimuli, (6) acute excessive and seemingly illogical anxiety, (7) loss or congenital lack of speech or failure to develop language competencies beyond a level appropriate to an earlier stage, (8) distortion in motility patterns, and (9) a background of serious retardation in which isolated areas of normal, near-normal or exceptional intellectual function or skills may appear.

Classification of Chronic Psychosis

- Autistic psychoses
  - Early infantile autism (Kanner, 1943)
  - Symbiotic Psychosis (Mahler, 1952)
- Schizophrenia
  - Simple
  - Paranoid
  - Acute undifferentiated

Kanner (1943, 1965) studied a specific group of psychotic children and described the clinical entity of infantile autism. These children are characterized by (1) inability to relate in normal ways to people and situations from very early infancy—preference for isolation and inanimate objects, (2) unusual language development—speech not used for purposes of communication, (3) behavior governed by an anxiously obsessive desire for maintenance of sameness and (4) a relatively normal physical appearance, with an apparently good cognitive potential.

Although autism occurs frequently in the first-born male, no clear relationship to birth order has been demonstrated. Most authors do agree, however, that autism occurs more frequently in males than in females, with the male:female ratio from 2:1 to 4.5:1. Some authors limit the diagnosis of autism to children manifesting autistic behavior from birth. Other investigators include cases with onset prior to age 3, following periods of normal development. The age of onset has been suggested as a basis for classification, with the diagnosis of infantile autism limited to patients with onset before age 2, that of childhood schizophrenia applied to patients with the onset after age 8, and patients with onset and regression between 3 and 8 years of age considered to be a heterogeneous group of organic psychotics.

In children with symbiotic psychosis, one finds a history of extreme mutual dependency between the child and the mother. The child may relate quite well to the mother and talk with her but is very withdrawn, anxious and afraid in the presence of other people and has no friends. Such a child is very immature emotionally and frequently has a thought disorder.

Rank (1955) described a group labeled "atypical children," stating that the essential feature of atypical development consisted of "ego fragmentation," i.e., individual components of the ego of the infant and young child do not develop in a coherent and concerted fashion because of complications in the parent/child relationship.

Etiology

The etiology of psychoses includes a whole gamut of contributing factors, including heredity, prenatal and postnatal insults, metabolic abnormalities and environmental influences. It is generally accepted that there exists some type of potential (hereditary, metabolic or as a result of brain damage) that predisposes these children to react more adversely to abnormal environmental influences. The complex interaction of these factors frequently leads to the development and maintenance of psychotic behavior (Hingtgen and Bryson, 1972).

An increased incidence of a variety of prenatal, perinatal and postnatal abnormalities in psychotic children supports the hypothesis that at least a subgroup of these children is organically damaged. Although gross physical stigmata have not been demonstrated, physical and metabolic abnormalities have been encountered in psychotic children with greater than normal frequency. Several studies have found psychotic children significantly below normal in weight, height and bone age. These differences could not be explained on the basis of diet or social class. Other studies have also reported primitive postural responses and decreased muscle tone in the majority of schizophrenic children.

A large number of psychotic children manifest signs of minimal brain dysfunction, including language dysfunction, perceptual motor deficits and some degree of fine and gross motor coordination difficulty. Autistic children seem to have a neurologically based language dysfunction, which seriously interferes with the acquisition of expressive speech and abstract language competence. Several studies have suggested that many psychotic children tend to make little use of the distance receptors of vision and hearing and make relatively greater use of the proximal receptors of touch, taste and smell. Because both vision and hearing are so directly involved in communication and most other higher-order adaptive acts, it is hypothesized that the receptor preferences of psychotic children are based upon some disorder in the visual and auditory systems.

Electroencephalographic studies indicate that a larger number of psychotic children than control group subjects demonstrate significantly more neuropathologic signs, such as paroxysmal spike-and-wave complexes, a low-voltage, irregular activity without any established rhythm and lack of phasic inhibition of the auditorily evoked response during the rapid eye movement (REM) stage of sleep. Of course, not all psychotic children have abnormal EEGs. Nor do these abnormal findings suggest any one specific type of organicity. A thorough neurologic examination, with appropriate follow-up tests, is indicated for all cases of childhood psychosis.

Galvanic skin response is reported to be uniformly lower in psychotic children when compared with normal children, regardless of the stimulus modality tested. Metabolic studies reveal minor to moderate degrees of metabolic imbalance in some psychotic children. The most dramatic alterations, appearing in the pituitary gland, consist of reduced secretions of gonadotropins, corticotropin, and thyrotropin. The severity of endocrine imbalance appeared to be positively related to the degree of psychotic disturbance. Several biochemical abnormalities have been reported, such as higher platelet serotonin in autistic children and decreased serotonin uptake by platelets of schizophrenic children.

Unfortunately, none of the biochemical parameters studied to date, including the biogenic amines, the pink spot, the mauve factor, bufotenin, histamine, serum factors, chromosomal abnormalities, endocrinologic changes or other metabolic factors, have been shown to be causally related to the etiology of any of the childhood psychoses. Many of the investigations suffer from inadequate experimental design, from lack of rigorous control of such relevant variables as diet, hospitalization, stress and medication or from the use of insensitive or nonspecific chemical techniques. In addition, the number of subjects has frequently been small. However, a growing consensus is developing among investigators that the most likely cause of childhood psychosis will be found in some form of multiply determined brain abnormality. As a consequence, there is a renewed interest in autopsy studies.

Environmental theories of childhood psychosis emphasize abnormalities in the family relationship, problems in early communication and traumatic events. The parents of psychotic children are often described as cold, aloof, introverted and mechanical in their relationships with people, but when actual comparisons have been made—either with the general population or other clinical groups—data have proved inconclusive. Although some investigators have reported that the parents of psychotic children are of higher intellectual, educational and socioeconomic status than parents of other clinical groups, other investigators have found no differences. There is no evidence of increased paternal age, and evidence regarding maternal age is mixed. Findings of a lowered incidence of broken homes and of an unelevated or lower incidence of familial psychosis than in other emotionally disturbed groups are fairly conclusive. However, a higher incidence of nonpsychotic affective disturbances has been reported in the families of psychotic children.

Although many clinicians have speculated about psychopathology in the parents of psychotic children, there have been relatively few objective investigations of this matter. Moreover, results of the studies which have been conducted are inconsistent. The conception of a schizophrenogenic or refrigerated, mechanical mother who produces psychotic children is not well supported.

In symbiotic psychosis, an abnormally close relationship between the child and the mother is implied. There are, however, indications that in at least some cases, these children may be predisposed to excessive dependency by unknown physical conditions. Thus, an abnormally close relationship may satisfy the dependency needs of both the child and the mother.

Management of Chronic Psychoses

Many patients may recover completely from acute psychotic episodes that are associated with organic conditions. A few patients may also completely recover from an acute episode of functional psychosis. The majority of patients with acute functional psychosis and some patients with acute organic psychosis, however, do not recover completely and continue to suffer from a residual or chronic type of psychosis, accompanied by a lower level of social, vocational and emotional adjustment as compared with the adjustment levels in these areas prior to the acute episode. Many of these patients may require periodic administration of antipsychotic drugs to alleviate their anxiety, delusions and hallucinations.

In some children, psychosis is an insidious process. These children are very quiet and withdrawn from their early years. They are shy, isolated and have few friends. They often play with much younger children to whom they are good companions. Any new activity or new situation makes them feel very anxious, and it takes them a long time to become accustomed to new situations. In school, they complete their assignments without much difficulty and thus frequently escape the teacher's attention until they are asked to participate in group activities or are called upon to read in front of the class. They then become highly anxious and are frequently unable to take part in these activities.

The management of children with chronic psychosis requires a comprehensive plan aimed at promoting social, emotional and educational development. These children should attend a regular school if possible. The teacher should be apprised of the child's condition and advised not to push the child into group participation activities and situations. Placement in a special school may be necessary if the child is unable to keep up academically with his classmates, or if he becomes highly anxious in the regular classroom.

The parents should be helped through counseling to understand the child's difficulties, especially difficulties with social relationships. They can do a great deal to promote interaction with peers by gradually introducing the child to new peers and new situations.

Many of these children require psychotherapy of several years' duration. The goals of psychotherapy include developing an anxiety-free relationship with the child, helping him to understand his fears and inhibitions and aiding him in overcoming them. This final goal, however, is rarely achieved in therapy, and most of these children grow up to be shy and withdrawn adults.

Stressful life events, such as starting school, parental separation and the beginning of adolescence, are likely to cause acute episodes of severe anxiety, which may trigger acute delusions, hallucinations and bizarre behavior. Such episodes are treated by modifying the environment to reduce the anxiety and by the administration of antipsychotic drugs (as described in the section on the management of acute psychoses).

Children with infantile autism are frequently identified and diagnosed before the age of 2 or 3. An intensive program of training is instituted as soon as the diagnosis is made. These programs are usually organized by special nursery schools and consist of structured play and educational activities in which children are gently pushed to participate. Parents are counseled to spend time with the children at home in similar types of activities. Antipsychotic medications (e.g., phenothiazine, Haldol) can sometimes reduce the child's inhibition and improve his participation in various activities.

Children with symbiotic psychosis require special treatment programs in which both the child and the mother jointly participate. The mother's presence is gradually reduced over a period of several months after other adults have developed a positive relationship with the child. The mother and the child may require psychotherapy of several years' duration to sever their symbiotic ties and to develop a more normal relationship.

REFERENCES

Bender, L.: Childhood schizophrenia. Symposium (1955). Its recognition, description and treatment, Am. J. Orthopsychiatry 26:499, 1956.

Creak, M.: Schizophrenic syndrome in childhood. Progress report of a working party, Br. Med. J. 2:889, 1961.

Hingtgen, J. N., and Bryson, C. Q.: Recent developments in the study of early childhood psychoses: Infantile autism, childhood schizophrenia and related disorders, Schizophrenia Bull. 5:8, 1972.

Kanner, L.: Autistic disturbances of affective contact, Nervous Child 2:217, 1943.

Kanner, L.: Infantile autism and schizophrenia, Behav. Sci. 10:412, 1965.

Lotter, V.: Epidemiology of autistic conditions in young children: I. Prevalence, Soc.'Psychiatry 1:124, 1966.

Mahler, M. S.: On child psychosis and schizophrenia: Autistic and symbiotic infantile psychoses, Psychoanal. Study Child 7:286, 1952.

Nikolovski, O. T., and Fernandez, J. V.: Report 68: Capgras syndrome as an aftermath of chickenpox encephalitis, Psychiatric Opinion 15:39, 1978.

Potter, H. W.:'Schizophrenia in children, Am. J. Psychiatry 89:1253, 1933.

Rank, B.: Intensive study and treatment of preschool children who show marked personality deviations, or "atypical development," and their parents, in Caplan, C. (ed.): Emotional Problems of Early Childhood (New York: Basic Books, Inc., 1955).

Treffert, D. A.: The epidemiology of infantile autism, Arch. Gen. Psychiatry 22:431, 1970.

9/Drug Treatment of Acute Psychiatric Conditions

THERE ARE AT LEAST 60 drugs in psychiatry that are useful in the treatment of mental disturbances. They have been classified in various ways: major or minor tranquilizers, ataractics, neuroleptics, psychotropics. In recent years, the tendency has been to classify these drugs as antipsychotic, antidepressant and antianxiety agents on the basis of their predominant clinical effect. Few of these drugs have been used previously to treat children, since there is a lack of sufficient experimental data. It is important, however, to become familiar with some of these drugs, since they are now being used to treat the emotional disorders of children.

Table 9–1 provides the classification of common drugs presently used in psychiatry.

Antipsychotic Drugs

These drugs have truly revolutionized the treatment of institutionalized mental patients since the mid-1950s. Many large mental hospitals have reduced their census sharply downward, and some of them have closed entirely. The management of violent and aggressive patients has become more humane. Since the clinical features of psychoses vary from patient to patient, it is important to recognize the differences among the various classes of antipsychotic drugs in order to match each patient with the best available drug.

Phenothiazines

Most of the drugs available within this class are equally effective as antipsychotic agents. However, there are differences among the 3 subclasses with regard to their potency, side effects and other pharmacologic properties that make them differentially useful for specific patients. As is evident in Table 9–1, one needs higher dosage levels in the aliphatic and piperidine groups than in the piperazine group to achieve the same degree of clinical effectiveness. The aliphatics have more marked sedative-hypnotic, motor-inhibiting, mood-dampening actions than do the piperazines, which are likely to be activating and more stimulating. The aliphatics are

TABLE 9–1.—DRUGS USED IN PSYCHIATRY

GENERIC NAME	REGISTERED TRADE NAME	ESTIMATED EQUIVALENT DOSE (MG)	TOTAL DAILY DOSE (MG)
	ANTIPSYCHOTIC DRUGS		
Phenothiazines			
Aliphatic group			
Chlorpromazine	Thorazine	100	50–1,000
Promazine	Sparine	100	25–1,000
Triflupromazine	Vesprin	25	50–150
Piperidine group			
Thioridazine	Mellaril	100	50–800
Mesoridazine	Serentil	50	50–400
Piperacetazine	Quide	10	10–160
Piperazine group			
Perphenazine	Trilafon	8	12–64
Prochlorperazine	Compazine	15	10–150
Thiopropazate	Dartal	10	10–100
Trifluoperazine	Stelazine	5	5–30
Acetophenazine	Tindal	20	40–80
Butaperazine	Repoise	10	15–100
Carphenazine	Proketazine	25	25–400
Fluphenazine	Permitil, Prolixin	2	1–20
Butyrophenones			
Haloperidol	Haldol	2	2–15
Thioxanthenes			
Chlorprothixene	Taractan	100	25–600
Thiothixene	Navane	4	5–30
	ANTIDEPRESSANT DRUGS		
Tricyclic group			
Iminodibenzyl derivatives			
Imipramine	Tofranil		75–150
Desipramine	Norpramine		30–150
Trimepramine	Surmontil		75–300
Dibenzocycloheptene derivatives			
Amitriptyline	Elavil		75–150
Nortriptyline	Aventyl		75–200
Protriptyline	Vivactil		10–30
Dibenzoxepin derivatives			
Doxepin	Sinequan		50–400
Monoamine oxidase inhibitors			
Hydrazine derivatives			
Isocarboxazid	Marplan		30–50
Phenelzine	Nardil		10–75
Nialamide	Niamide		12.5–200
Monohydrazine derivatives			
Pargyline	Eutonyl		25–75
Tranylcypromine	Parnate		10–30
Lithium carbonate	Lithane, Lithonate		750–2,500

TABLE 9–1.—*Continued*

GENERIC NAME	REGISTERED TRADE NAME	ESTIMATED EQUIVALENT DOSE (MG.)	TOTAL DAILY DOSE (MG)
ANTIANXIETY DRUGS			
Benzodiazepines			
Chlordiazepoxide	Librium		10–100
Diazepam	Valium		6–40
Chlorazepate	Tranxene		7.5–60
Oxazepam	Serax		30–120
Lorazepam	Ativan		1–6
Substituted propanediols			
Meprobamate	Equanil, Miltown		600–1,200
Tybamate	Solacen		750 1,200
Phenaglycodol	Ultran		800–1,200
Oxanamide	Quiactin		800–1,600
Diphenylmethane derivatives			
Hydroxyzine	Atarax, Vistaril		30–100
Benactyzine	Phobex, Suavitil		3–9
Captodiamine	Suvren		300–400
Azacylonol	Frenquel		60–300
Buclizine	Softran		100–300
CENTRAL NERVOUS SYSTEM STIMULANT DRUGS			
Racemicamphetamine	Benzedrine		5–30
Dextroamphetamine	Dexedrine		5–30
Methylphenidate	Ritalin		5–15
Methamphetamine	Methedrine, Desoxyn		2.5–20
Deanol	Deaner		25–75
Pipradol	Meratran		1–7.5

more likely to produce hematologic, hepatotoxic, hypotensive, autonomic or photosensitivity reactions than are the piperazines. The piperazines, on the other hand, are more likely to produce extrapyramidal side effects and occasional hypertension. On the basis of these differences, it is recommended that the drugs of the aliphatic and piperidine groups be given to more agitated, hyperactive patients, while drugs in the piperazine group be given to withdrawn, anergic patients.

Other Antipsychotic Drugs

The thioxanthenes and the butyrophenones are as effective antipsychotics as are the phenothiazines. They differ, however, in their toxicity and untoward effects. As a class, the thioxanthenes produce few hepatotoxic, hematologic and photosensitivity reactions but are more likely to produce extrapyramidal side effects. Similarly, haloperidol, a butyrophenone, is a potent antipsychotic agent, whose sedative and hypnotic effect is of much smaller magnitude than that of the phenothiazines. It is reported, however, to have the highest potential of all antipsychotic drugs for inducing extrapyramidal side effects. It may be used as a substitute for phenothiazine in patients with jaundice or in patients with skin reactions to phenothiazines.

MECHANISM OF ACTION.—Chlorpromazine differs from barbiturates in its effects on the brain stem reticular formation. Electrical potentials in the cortex following direct stimulation of the reticular formation are not affected by chlorpromazine but are depressed by barbiturates. However, potentials recorded in the reticular formation following peripheral stimulation are considerably reduced by chlorpromazine. Chlorpromazine may thus have an action related to the inflow of sensory information to the reticular formation.

Inhibition of dopamine functions in the central nervous system appears to be a common basic property of antipsychotic drugs. The mesolimbic and nigrostriatal portions of the dopaminergic system are probably the main targets for the mental and the extrapyramidal actions, respectively, of these drugs. Increased concentrations of dopamine induced by amphetamines or dopa may lead to a disturbance mimicking paranoid schizophrenia. This lends further support for a key role of dopamine in mental functions.

Chlorpromazine produces interneuronal block in the spinal cord by a supraspinal action. It has a powerful effect on the emetic chemoreceptor trigger zone in the medulla and abolishes vomiting due to apomorphine. It also lowers body temperature. It has a considerable alpha-adrenergic blocking effect and, by virtue of this and its effect upon the hypothalamus, tends to lower blood pressure. It causes peripheral vasodilation, which raises skin temperature and also increases heat loss. The normal vasoconstrictor mechanisms are impaired, and the blood pressure falls when the subject rises to the upright position (orthostatic hypotension).

The basic schizophrenic symptoms, such as thought disorder, delusions and hallucinations, are less affected than tension and excitement, and in this sense antipsychotic drugs are not truly curative. Nevertheless, the psychotic symptoms are greatly moderated and may even disappear, although patients frequently relapse within a few weeks after medication is stopped.

ADMINISTRATION.—Chlorpromazine is usually given by mouth, but it can be administered by deep intramuscular injection and by suppository.

Intramuscular injection may cause a fall in blood pressure and fainting. The oral dose varies over a wide range, from 30 mg for a mild emotional upset to doses of 1–2 gm per day in hospitalized, aggressive, psychotic patients. The smaller dose is of questionable value. In outpatient treatment of children, dosage is gradually increased over a period of several weeks until maximum improvement is evident. This maximum dosage is continued for about 2 weeks, then is gradually reduced to the lowest effective maintenance level.

Maintenance therapy should be accompanied by periodic checks of the plasma levels of the psychoactive drugs, along with determinations of complete blood count and liver function tests. There is little in the literature on the relationship between plasma levels of psychoactive drugs and their clinical effectiveness. Garver and associates (1977) reported a definite relationship between plasma levels of chlorpromazine and therapeutic response. The relationship, however, was a nonlinear one, that is, there was an optimal plasma level of chlorpromazine below which there was less or no therapeutic response. This phenomenon has been referred to as the "therapeutic window." Rivera-Calimlim et al. (1973) also concluded that there was a nonlinear relationship, that is, patients who did not improve clinically showed low plasma levels of chlorpromazine, while those who improved significantly had plasma levels 5 to 10 times higher. No plasma levels of antipsychotic drugs effective in children have been reported.

Phenothiazines do not cause psychic dependence and do not produce tolerance or addiction. Abrupt withdrawal of high-dose therapy is not recommended, however, as in some cases symptoms resembling those of physical dependence, such as gastritis, nausea, vomiting, dizziness and trembling, may appear.

Chlorpromazine is well absorbed from the gastrointestinal tract and is distributed to all tissues. It is excreted in the urine largely as glucuronide or as chlorpromazine sulfoxide. It is eliminated slowly from the body, and in patients medicated for long periods, traces of the drug or its metabolites may be found in the urine up to several months after its discontinuance.

TOXIC EFFECTS.—The toxic effects of antipsychotic drugs are of two kinds: effects of overdosage and allergic hypersensitivity reactions.

The main symptoms of overdosage are sedation, hypotension and extrapyramidal effects. Most patients experience some degree of drowsiness, but tolerance to the sedative effect develops after a few weeks. The patient usually sleeps well at night, although he may experience vivid dreams.

Extrapyramidal side effects are frequently reported during the first few weeks of treatment. In most patients, these reactions involve Parkinson-like symptoms. Other types of reactions, such as motor restlessness, dystonia, akathisia, hyperreflexia, opisthotonos and oculogyric crisis, are reported far less frequently. Severe extrapyramidal reactions have been reported to occur at relatively low doses. However, the occurrence and severity of most extrapyramidal symptoms are dose related and occur at relatively high doses and disappear or become less severe when the dose is reduced.

Persistent tardive dyskinesia may develop after long-term drug therapy. It is characterized by slow, involuntary, writhing movements of the tongue, mouth or face and often other parts of the body as well. Sucking, chewing, licking and blowing movements are the more commonly affected motor activities. The risk appears to be greater in elderly patients on long-term therapy, or symptoms may appear after drug therapy has been discontinued. The symptoms of tardive dyskinesia are persistent and in some patients appear to be irreversible.

There is no known effective treatment for tardive dyskinesia; antiparkinsonism agents usually do not alleviate the symptoms of this syndrome. It has been reported that fine vermicular movements of the tongue may be an early sign of the syndrome, and if medication is stopped at this time, the syndrome may not develop.

All antipsychotic drugs are likely to cause some changes in EKG, with phenothiazines of the piperidine and aliphatic groups producing EKG changes more frequently than phenothiazines of other groups. The alterations consist of flattening, notching or lowering of the T waves, sometimes associated with a small lengthening of the Q-T interval. Apparently, these changes are benign and represent a modification of ventricular repolarization. They disappear when the drug is reduced in dose or discontinued. They can be abolished during treatment by coadministration of potassium salts. Whether these changes can lead to a cardiac arrythmia cannot be conclusively stated. However, in doses exceeding the recommended maximum limit, drugs of the thioridazine group have allegedly induced heart block and ventricular fibrillation.

A reaction, probably allergic, that occurs in a small percentage of patients treated with antipsychotic drugs, often during the first few weeks of treatment, is obstructive jaundice due to cholestatic hepatitis. This complication necessitates discontinuance of the drug. It is sometimes possible after the jaundice has cleared to resume medication with another antipsychotic drug. In this case, however, dangerous blood dyscrasias may also occur.

Antiparkinsonism Drugs

These drugs are used to relieve the symptoms of parkinsonism and the extrapyramidal side effects often induced by antipsychotic drugs. They

TABLE 9–2.—ANTIPARKINSONISM DRUGS

GENERIC NAME	TRADE NAME	DAILY DOSE (ADULT)
Benztropine	Cogentin	0.5–6 mg
Procyclidine	Kemadrin	5–15 mg
Biperiden	Akineton	2–8 mg
Trihexyphenidyl	Artane, Tremin	1–10 mg
Amantadine Hydrochloride	Symmetrel	100–300 mg
Cycrimine	Pagitane	5–20 mg

usually act by diminishing muscle tone and involuntary movements. Table 9–2 lists some of the common antiparkinsonism drugs used in psychiatry.

These drugs can be divided into four groups:

1. Synthetic anticholinergics, such as trihexyphenidyl, biperiden, cycrimine and procyclidine. These drugs produce atropine-like untoward effects, such as dryness of the mouth, blurred vision, dizziness and dysuria. Trihexyphenidyl is available in tablets of 2 and 5 mg, time-released capsules of 5 mg, and elixir, 2 mg/5ml. Dosage ranges from 1 mg initially to a maximum of 20 mg daily.

2. Antihistamines, such as diphenhydramine (Benadryl) and orphenadrine (Norflex). These drugs are not as effective as the anticholinergics but produce fewer atropine-like untoward effects. On the other hand they produce considerable drowsiness.

3. Drugs with both anticholinergic and antihistaminic properties. Benztropine (Cogentin) is the major representative of this class. Its pharmacologic properties resemble those of atropine not only with regard to untoward effects but also from the standpoint of duration of action, which is long.

4. Miscellaneous drugs, including amantadine and dextroamphetamine. Amantadine is an antiviral agent. Its mode of action is not understood, although there are some experimental findings suggestive of an amantadine-dopamine interaction. Adverse effects of amantadine include hyperexcitability, slurred speech, ataxia, insomnia, and gastrointestinal disturbances. Convulsions have occurred after the administration of excessive doses. The initial dose for adults is 100 mg once daily for 5–7 days.

Antiparkinsonism drugs should not be used routinely for prophylaxis, with antipsychotic drugs. Data suggest that not only do they afford no protection but that they may be detrimental to the patient—by increasing the side effects and by inhibiting the actions of the antipsychotic drugs. Trihexephenidyl has been shown to significantly decrease the serum level of chlorpromazine as well as to retard or reverse the clinical improvement chlorpromazine may produce. If used to treat extrapyramidal side effects, antiparkinsonism drugs should be given just once a day and should be administered continuously for 3–4 months in the majority of cases. Extrapyramidal symptoms tend to recur if the drugs are given for fewer than 3–4 months, and giving them for more than 4 months does not provide any benefit to patients.

Antiparkinsonism medication can effectively alleviate the dystonia, rigidity, akathesia and rabbit syndrome movements associated with the antipsychotics. The rabbit syndrome involves involuntary puckering of the mouth and flaring of the nostrils. It usually occurs in middle-aged patients and is not related to tardive dyskinesia.

Use of Antipsychotic Drugs in Children

Since the early 1970s, phenothiazines have been used to manage behavioral problems in mentally retarded, brain-damaged, cerebral palsied and emotionally disturbed children. Heuyer et al. (1953) reported a beneficial effect of chlorpromazine in calming children who had severe outbursts of excitement. Freedman et al. (1955) found that chlorpromazine was effective in the treatment of schizophrenic children who were hyperactive. Similarly, Hunt et al. (1956) showed that hyperactivity and social relatedness were consistently improved in schizophrenic children by the administration of chlorpromazine. Fish (1960) reported on the use of other phenothiazines as they became available, such as prochlorperazine, trifluoperazine and perphenazine. She reported a beneficial, stimulating effect of trifluoperazine on withdrawn, hypoactive, schizophrenic children. Shaw et al. (1963) reported that four of the phenothiazines—trifluoperazine, fluphenazine, trifluophenazine and thioridazine—were all effective in relieving symptoms of anxiety, excitability, aggressiveness and impulsivity in a heterogeneous group of children living in a residential treatment center.

Greenberg et al. (1972) compared the effects of chlorpromazine, dextroamphetamines, hydroxyzine and placebo in a group of children with the hyperkinetic syndrome. They found that both chlorpromazine and dextroamphetamine were significantly better than placebo, hydroxyzine was generally ineffective, and dextroamphetamine produced either strongly favorable or strongly unfavorable reactions, with fewer of the latter.

Saletu et al. (1974) showed that thioxanthine, compared to placebo, produced a significant and persistent improvement, beginning in the second week, of motor activity, speech, social relationships, affect and behavior disturbance.

Haloperidol has been reported to be the most effective treatment for Gilles de la Tourette syndrome.

Antianxiety Drugs

Anxiety is perceived as a pervasive feeling of apprehension about some unspecified future threat to self-esteem. This threat may be based on a memory of a past threat triggered by some unrecognized present stimulus. The memory may trigger the emotions and the somatic responses of the past fearful state. The somatic manifestations of anxiety are many and affect virtually all organ systems. Some of the most common are fatigue, dizziness, palpitation, indigestion, bowel disturbances, headaches, muscle aches, insomnia, excessive perspiration, trembling of hands or voice and other signs of nervous tension.

Benzodiazepines are by far the most commonly prescribed class of antianxiety drugs in the world. General practitioners account for the single largest block of prescriptions for these drugs, followed in decreasing numbers of prescriptions written by internists, psychiatrists, surgeons, osteopaths, obstetricians, gynecologists and neurologists. However, on a rate-of-prescribing basis, psychiatrists, neurologists and internists head the list, with general practitioners and other specialists trailing behind. Diagnostic categories treated with these drugs include anxiety reactions, circulatory disorders of various kinds (e.g., hypertension), digestive disorders, tension headaches, back pain and surgical aftercare cases. A careful scrutiny of the data indicates that the reason for prescribing the benzodiazepines was remarkably similar across specialties (NDTI, 1975). Tranquilization was the chief action desired, being sought in 45–67% of the prescriptions. Sedation-hypnosis was the second most common action desired (8–29% of uses). The only impressive difference across specialties lay in the desired action of skeletal muscle relaxation, which was sought by 1–8% of all specialty groups except for surgeons and neurologists, who sought this action in 30% and 22% of uses, respectively.

Glycol derivatives, such as meprobamate, were the first antianxiety agents. Their lesser degree of effectiveness in the treatment of anxiety has led to their replacement by the benzodiazepines.

The sedative effects of some of the antihistamines (diphenhydramine and hydroxyzine) have been utilized to relieve anxiety in young children. Diphenhydramine has been used as a mild sedative and hypnotic in the treatment of children for decades. The efficacy of hydroxyzine (Atarax) in the management of anxiety is less clear. Although benzodiazepines are being widely used in children and adolescents, data with regard to their efficacy and indications are not fully available. Psychiatric indications for the use of the benzodiazepines in children include anxiety, psychosomatic disorders, phobias and explosive temper with frequent aggressive outbursts.

Benzodiazepines

The popularity of benzodiazepines depends a great deal upon their wide range of actions and their lesser degree of toxicity when compared to antipsychotic drugs. Benzodiazepines, however, possess little antipsychotic effect but instead cause muscle relaxation and have antianxiety and anticonvulsant effects and sedative and hypnotic effects. They are capable of calming aggressive animals when given in smaller doses than that required for a muscle relaxant effect.

An important use of the benzodiazepines is in the management of alcohol withdrawal symptoms and delirium tremens. They calm the patient promptly and effectively, have anticonvulsant activity and are unlikely to create physical or psychological dependence.

PHARMACOKINETICS.—Chlorazepate is hydrolyzed in the stomach to an active metabolite, desmethyldiazepam (DMDZ). Desmethyldiazepam is also the first major active metabolite of diazepam, following its demethylation by the liver. Thus, chlorazepate and diazepam, given orally, are both initially metabolized to DMDZ. The rate and the extent of the hydrolysis of chlorazepate to DMDZ seem to depend on gastric acidity. The completeness of absorption depends upon the extent of hydrolysis. As the pH in the upper gastrointestinal tract approaches 7, the hydrolysis half-life becomes longer, suggesting that gastric emptying must occur before a substantial degree of hydrolysis takes place. Patients with achlorhydria or those taking antacids may not produce and absorb clinically useful amounts of DMDZ following chlorazepate dosage. Absorption of chlordiazepoxide also appears to be delayed with concomitant use of antacids. The lipophilic nature of diazepam may also lead to malabsorption of this drug if it is ingested with mineral oil.

With the exception of the hydrolysis of chlorazepate to DMDZ in the stomach, the major site of biotransformation of the benzodiazepines is the liver. Demethylation and/or hydroxylation are important steps in the biotransformation of chlordiazepoxide and diazepam. Liver disease, especially in alcoholics and the elderly, may influence these processes. Findings suggest that elimination of oxazepam, which is already 3-hydroxylated and does not undergo demethylation, is not impaired either in alcoholics or in elderly individuals (Schull et al., 1976).

The effects of age on the apparent elimination half-life have more potential clinical importance. The chlordiazepoxide elimination half-life in an elderly group as a whole was more than 60% longer than in young volunteers. Administrators of these drugs should take this into account to avoid unwanted effects in the elderly.

Studies (Shader and Greenblatt, 1977) suggest that chlordiazepoxide and diazepam are better absorbed from the gastrointestinal tract than from intramuscular injections, which result in delayed and possibly incomplete absorption of the parent drug, as well as delayed appearance of its active metabolite. However, intramuscular administration of lorazepam, a 3-hydroxybenzodiazepine derivative similar in structure to oxazepam, may lead to rapid absorption of the drug from the injection site and prompt clinical effects.

MECHANISM OF ACTION.—Benzodiazepines are clinically useful in the treatment of anxiety, seizures and muscular spasms. The myriad effects of these drugs are probably mediated by several distinct mechanisms. Neurotransmitters implicated in mediation processes include norepinephrine, serotonin, and gamma aminobutyric acid (GABA) and glycine.

Norepinephrine antagonizes the depressant effect of oxazepam (Stein et al., 1973). This observation suggests that the depressant action of benzodiazepines may be mediated at least in part by reduction of noradrenergic activity. Similarly, serotonin has been found to decrease the anxiety-reducing effect of oxazepam, suggesting that sertonin systems may be implicated in the anxiety-reducing actions of benzodiazepines.

Gamma-aminobutyric acid is one of the two major inhibitory transmitters in the brain. Between 25% and 40% of all synapses throughout the brain use GABA as their neurotransmitter (Iversen and Bloom, 1972). Compared with GABA, the biogenic amines are like trace elements in neurotransmission. It has been estimated that norepinephrine and dopamine each account for only 1% of the brain synapses, that the proportion of serotonin synapses is substantially lower and that the number of cholinergic synapses is probably only 5–10% of total brain synapses. GABA is contained in the short interneurons as well as in neurons with lengthy axons that connect distant regions of the brain. It has been suggested that benzodiazepines cause direct binding of GABA to physiologic synaptic receptors. The rate of synthesis and release of GABA may also be influenced by benzodiazepines.

Besides having functions in general metabolism, glycine is an inhibitory neurotransmitter in the brain stem and spinal cord, at which locations it accounts for a total of 25% of all synapses (Stein et al., 1973). Benzodiazepines seem to compete with glycine for receptor binding.

Almost all the actions of the benzodiazepines currently available for review seem to be compatible with a theory of GABA-mediated potentiation of presynaptic and postsynaptic inhibition, including the moderate decreases in biochemical indices of activity in catecholamine, acetylcholine and serotonin neurons. However, the emergence of new neurotransmitters, such as substance P (Takahashi et al., 1974) and the morphine-like peptides, suggests the need for prudence and caution before accepting monolithic explanations of the actions of the benzodiazepines.

The muscle relaxation effect of the benzodiazepines is exerted partly at the spinal level through inhibition of polysynaptic spinal reflexes. The main effect is probably at the brain stem level and caused by depression of neurons that exaggerate the discharge of gamma motor neurons during tension and anxiety states.

The antianxiety effect of the benzodiazepines appears to be mediated by the limbic system. Benzodiazepines do not act on the seizure focus itself but produce their anticonvulsant effect by inhibiting the spread of the seizure.

In common with other hypnotics, benzodiazepines shorten the relative duration of rapid eye movement sleep (REM), but rather less so than the barbiturates. They also seem to exhibit less REM rebound after withdrawal. A characteristic change in sleep pattern appears to be a reduction of the duration of slow wave sleep.

TOXIC EFFECTS.—Benzodiazepines are relatively nontoxic, and this is an important reason for their widespread use. They cause relatively little depression of the vital centers of the medulla. The incidence of successful suicide with these drugs is not reported.

Their most common untoward effects are drowsiness, lethargy, muscle weakness and ataxia. Large doses may cause fainting. These effects are particularly likely to occur in elderly patients. When given to psychotic patients, chlordiazepoxide may paradoxically cause attacks of rage and confusion. Because of their sedative effects, these drugs are dangerous to drivers, especially in combination with alcohol.

Diphenylmethane Derivatives

Drugs in this group may be termed "sedative-autonomic," and unlike other antianxiety drugs, they affect the peripheral autonomic nervous system. They are not popular drugs, perhaps because they create feelings of restlessness and mental fuzziness as well as having bothersome peripheral side effects, such as dry mouth and blurred vision.

Diphenylmethane derivatives include certain antihistaminic and anticholinergic drugs. Hydroxyzine and buclizine are antihistaminic and anticholinergic agents; benactyzine is an anticholinergic drug. Hydroxyzine produces drowsiness and has antihistaminic and antiemetic properties, in addition to an antianxiety effect. It has a slight atropine-like action and a slight adrenergic blocking action and a mild quinidine-like effect. Benactyzine is basically an anticholinergic drug with many central nervous system actions, has atropine-like actions, produces mydriasis, inhibits salivation, is an antispasmodic and causes drowsiness. This drug is not popular as an antianxiety agent.

TOLERANCE AND PHYSICAL DEPENDENCE.—Tolerance to and physical dependence symptoms caused by antianxiety agents vary with the different groups of these drugs. Tolerance develops rapidly to meprobamate, with laboratory evidence indicating that the rate of hydroxylation of this drug doubles after a week of exposure. Tolerance to the benzodiazepines is slow to develop. Most drugs of the sedative-autonomic class do not readily produce tolerance. Development of physical dependence on chlordiazepoxide requires a high level of abuse (6 to 20 times the therapeutic dose). Withdrawal reactions are of much greater severity and intensity with meprobamate than with chlordiazepoxide and diazepam.

Antidepressant Drugs

Some of the most active cerebral stimulants belong to the group of sympathomimetic amines. The central effects of epinephrine are brief and are shown by apprehension and excitement. Ephedrine has a more prolonged central stimulant action. Amphetamine and related drugs have been used to overcome fatigue and depression.

Although the sympathomimetic drugs increase alertness and allay fatigue in normal human beings, they have been found to be of little value in the treatment of clinical depression. They tend to make the depressed more restless and agitated without lifting the lowered mood.

The newer antidepressants belonging to the tricyclic and the monoamine oxidase inhibitor groups counteract depression without producing overt stimulation. Tricyclic antidepressants have become the most widely used medications in the treatment of depression. These drugs include imipramine, amitriptyline, their demethylated metabolites, desipramine and nortriptyline, and some variants, such as protriptyline and doxepin. Monoamine oxidase inhibitors, after prolonged controversy, are making a comeback. The 2 drugs of this group still used as antidepressants are phenelzine and tranylcypromine (Parnate).

Tricyclic Antidepressants

The major effects of the tricyclic antidepressants are consequences of their antidepressant and anticholinergic actions. Minor effects are related to sedation, antihistaminic action and potentiation of the action of adrenergic drugs. They also have a quinidine-like effect on the heart.

After a delay of several days, the tricyclic compounds elevate the mood, increase alertness and improve appetite in large numbers of patients. Unfortunately, most studies of the efficacy of antidepressants have been done with heterogeneous populations of depressed individuals. Under such circumstances, it is not surprising that the differences between tricyclic antidepressants and placebos have sometimes been difficult to demonstrate. When these drugs have been studied in carefully selected patients with true endogenous depression, their worth has been proved. Most depression in children and adolescents is obviously reactive to personal or environmental difficulties or losses in the family or friends. They are best worked through psychologically. A classic endogenous depression with a strong family history, a history of past episodes and marked physical or somatic symptoms, such as loss of appetite or psychomotor retardation, are clear indications for tricyclic antidepressants. The presence of a precipitating cause does not rule out endogenous depression, but a discrepancy between the magnitude of the misfortune and the depressive reaction should raise this diagnostic possibility.

Anticholinergic actions are responsible for many side effects, but whether these are pertinent to the antidepressant effect is questionable.

Sedation may be considerable, and there is an increasing tendency to prescribing the tricyclic drugs in a single dose at bedtime. The antihistaminic action of these drugs is of no practical importance.

Tricyclics differ in their relative sedative and anticholinergic effects. Amitriptyline and doxepin are the most sedative, followed by imipramine and protriptyline. Amitriptyline clearly has the most cholinergic effect, followed by the others in somewhat the same order.

METABOLISM.—Tricyclics are well absorbed, although some degradation may occur in the gut or on passing through the liver. They are generally highly bound to plasma proteins, but a wide variation in degree of protein binding occurs between individuals. At the present time, it is not at all clear that monitoring plasma concentrations of these drugs will be clinically useful in helping the clinician to define an adequate therapeutic dose. These drugs are metabolized principally by ring hydroxylation and side-chain demethylation. The latter leads to active monodemethylated metabolites (secondary amines such as desipramine and nortriptyline), which invariably accumulate when patients are treated with the tertiary amines (such as amitriptyline and imipramine). The plasma disappearance rate is of fairly long duration, although exceedingly variable, suggesting the feasibility of a single daily dosage.

MECHANISM OF ANTIDEPRESSANT ACTION.—The antidepressant effect of tricyclic drugs is attributed primarily to their ability to block the active transport system by which released neurotransmitters are recaptured into the presynaptic nerve endings, the so-called amine pump. Tertiary amines, such as amitriptyline and imipramine, are thought to block the uptake of serotonin, whereas secondary amines, such as nortriptyline and desipramine, preferentially block the transport of norepinephrine. Of the tertiary amines, amitriptyline is less susceptible to metabolism to the active secondary amine metabolite than is imipramine. If one assumed that depression was mediated by decreased serotonergic transmission, amitriptyline would be the drug of choice. On the other hand, if depression were thought to be caused by decreased noradrenergic transmission, one of the secondary amines would be the drug of choice.

SIDE EFFECTS.—The anticholinergic action of the tricyclics causes symptoms, such as dryness of the mouth, blurred vision, constipation and urinary retention. Occasional disorientation and mental confusion may also be due to central anticholinergic effects.

Cardiovascular side effects include tachycardia, arrhythmias and prolongation of atrioventricular conduction time.

Tricyclics may negate the antihypertensive action of such commonly used drugs as quanethidine, methyldopa and clonidine.

Monoamine Oxidase Inhibitors

Historically, monoamine oxidase (MAO) inhibitors were the first of the new antidepressants to be introduced, but they have been largely displaced by the tricyclic antidepressants, which are less toxic and whose clinical effectiveness is better substantiated.

Most MAO inhibitors are slow-acting antidepressants. It may take more than a week of continuous therapy before some elevation of mood and central stimulation is experienced.

MECHANISM OF ACTION.—The destruction of catecholamines is brought about by 2 enzymes, monoamine oxidase and catechol-o-methyl transferase. MAO is widely distributed and is present in practically all tissues. It is an intracellular enzyme contained mainly in the mitochondria, which catalyzes the oxidative deamination of the side chain of catecholamine and serotonin.

Norepinephrine (NE) is believed to be stored in the brain in at least three compartments: a stable pool contained in granules combined with ATP, a more labile pool in granules not combined with ATP and a nongranular pool near the cell membrane from which NE is released by nerve stimulation. NE is actively accumulated in the storage granules but also continuously leaks out into the nongranular pool, where it is destroyed by MAO. MAO inhibitors produce an irreversible interaction with MAO. When MAO is administered to experimental animals, MAO inhibitors produce changes in catecholamine metabolism, and the amounts of NE and dopamine in the brain are increased. At the same time, the normal urinary degradation product (VMA) is diminished, and urinary metanephrine is increased.

The administration of MAO inhibitors produces similar changes in serotonin metabolism. The amount of serotonin in the brain is increased, the urinary excretion of its metabolite (5-hydroxyindol acetic acid) is diminished, while that of tryptamine is increased.

TOXIC EFFECTS.—The acute toxic effects of an overdose of MAO inhibitors are agitation, convulsions and collapse. Excessive stimulation, tremors, insomnia and orthostatic hypotension may also occur. A serious toxic effect which may occur early in the course of therapy is hepatocellular jaundice.

Because MAO inhibitors interact with a variety of enzymes in addition to MAO, they prevent the normal destruction of other drugs, which may thus rise to dangerous levels. Coma and death after normal doses of meperidine or barbiturates have occurred in patients receiving MAO inhibitors. Similarly, hypertensive crises have been reported after ingestion of certain foods, such as cheese (containing tyramine), in patients also receiving MAO inhibitors.

Lithium

In 1949, Cade instituted the study of the effects of lithium carbonate on psychotic behavior following the observation that lithium carbonate caused lethargy in guinea pigs. Since that time, lithium has been used to treat psychosis, depression and mania. So far, 2 clear indications for its use have emerged. Its use in the treatment of mania is fairly well established, and its use as a prophylactic in manic-depressive individuals to prevent the recurrence of mania, although fairly well accepted, has not been confirmed.

There have been only a few reported studies of the use of lithium in children. Frommer (1968) mentioned some improvement in the hypomanic behavior of 5–14-year-old children receiving lithium. Annell (1969) used lithium to treat children with a wide variety of behavioral symptoms, including typical mania and cyclic mood swings with variable results. Campbell et al. (1972), compared lithium with chlorpromazine in 10 severely disturbed children aged 3 to 6 years. There was a greater diminution of symptoms with chlorpromazine than with lithium. The majority of the studies of lithium in the treatment of children is inconclusive, and the results are highly variable. The symptom complex that seemed to have improved most with lithium included emotional excitement, explosiveness, impulsivity, aggressiveness and hyperactivity.

KINETICS OF LITHIUM.—Lithium is absorbed efficiently from the gastrointestinal tract. Less than 1% of the oral dose may appear in the stools. Peak concentrations in blood plasma occur 30 minutes after oral doses and are followed by a plateau for the next 12–24 hours. From one third to two thirds of a single oral dose is excreted in the urine in 6–12 hours. The remainder of the lithium is excreted slowly over a period of several days. The half-life of disappearance from the blood plasma is about 24 hours. Peak concentrations in cerebrospinal fluid (CSF) occur later than those in the blood plasma. The concentration achieved in CSF remains lower than the levels in the blood plasma. Also, the distribution of lithium ions in the brain is quite uneven.

MECHANISMS OF ACTION.—The exact mechanisms of the action of lithium in manic-depressive illness are not known. Several hypotheses have been advanced based on several lines of inquiry. Lithium is freely soluble and is more evenly distributed in the body water than is sodium or potassium and may substitute for each of them. As it is physically similar to magnesium and chemically similar to calcium, it may act like the latter cations in stabilizing the structure of proteins or membranes or in replacing magnesium as a cofactor in bioenergetic processes. In the central nervous system, lithium may interfere with neuronal conduction or carbohydrate metabolism. Another possible effect is interference with various hormone-activated adenyl cyclases. Alterations in body distribution of electrolytes and increased excretion of cyclic adenosine monophosphate (cyclic AMP) have been described as phenomena associated with mania.

Lithium is reported to decrease catecholaminergic transmission by accelerating presynaptic turnover of amines, inhibiting their release or decreasing receptor sensitivity.

The normal diurnal peak of serum cortisol levels at 6–8 A.M. may be shifted to the night during mania. Lithium tends to restore the normal diurnal rhythm.

CLINICAL USE.—As lithium is distributed freely in the body water and is not metabolized, the relationship of plasma concentrations to clinical effects is much more reliable than is the case with other drugs. During an acute manic episode in adults, the range of effective plasma concentration is reported to be 0.9–1.4 mEq/L. Maintenance doses for extended treatment can be one half to two thirds of these values. In children, much smaller doses are used. In Campbell and co-workers' study (1972), maximum tolerated doses of lithium carbonate by young children were 450–900 mg per day (blood levels of 0.25–1.19 mEq/L).

UNTOWARD EFFECTS.—Adverse reactions to lithium seem to be dose related. In adult patients, they are seldom encountered below 1.5 mEq/L plasma level. Mild to moderate toxic reactions may occur at levels from 1.5 to 2.5 mEq/L, and moderate to severe toxic reactions may be seen at levels from 2.0 to 2.5 mEq/L. Fine tremor, polyuria and mild thirst may occur during initial therapy for the acute manic phase and may persist throughout the treatment. Transient nausea and general discomfort may also appear during the first few days of lithium administration.

Diarrhea, vomiting, drowsiness, muscular weakness and lack of coordination may be early signs of lithium intoxication and require either a reduction of dose or complete cessation.

Other reported toxic effects include epileptiform seizures, slurred speech, blurred vision, albuminuria, glycosuria, diminished thyroid function, cardiac arrhythmia, hypotension and leukocytosis. Lithium may also produce reversible flattening, isoelectricity and inversion of T waves in electrocardiograms.

Campbell et al. (1972) reported untoward symptoms in young children who were given daily doses as low as 450 mg. The symptoms included subjective feelings of being "tired and miserable" or "feeling sick." At higher doses, children manifested difficulties in articulation, motor retardation, motor excitation, irritability and pallor.

REFERENCES

Annell, A. L.: Lithium in the treatment of children and adolescents, Acta Psychiatr. Scand. [Suppl] 207:19, 1969.

Cade, J. F.: Lithium salts in the treatment of psychotic excitement, Med. J. Aust. 36:349, 1949.

Campbell, M., Fish, B., David, R., et al.: Lithium and chlorpromazine: a controlled crossover study of hyperactive, severely disturbed young children, J. Autism Child. Schizo. 2:234, 1972.

Fish, B.: Drug therapy in child psychiatry: Pharmacological aspects, Compr. Psychiatry 1:212, 1960.

Freedman, A. M., Effron, A. S., and Bender, L.: Pharmacotherapy in children with psychiatric illness, J. Nerv. Ment. Dis. 122:479, 1955.

Frommer, E. A.: Depressive illness in childhood, Br. J. Psychiatry, [Special pub. 2]:117, 1968.

Garver, D. L., Dekirmenjian, H., Davis, J. M., et al.: Neuroleptic drug levels and therapeutic response: Preliminary observations with red blood cell-bound butaperazine, Am. J. Psychiatry 134:304, 1977.

Greenberg, L. M., Deens, M. A., and McMahon, A.: Effects of dextroamphetamine, chlorpromazine, and hydroxyzine on behavior and performance in hyperactive children, Am. J. Psychol. 129:532, 1972.

Heuyer, G., Gerard, G., and Galibert, J.: Traitement de l'excitation psychometrics chez l'enfant pare, Arch. Fr. Pediatr. 9:961, 1953.

Hunt, B. R., Frank, T., and Krush, T. P.: Chlorpromazine in the treatment of severe emotional disorders of childhood, J. Dis. Child. 9:268, 1956.

Iversen, L. L., and Bloom, F. E.: Studies on the uptake of ^{3}H-GABA and ^{3}H-

glycine in slices and homogenates of rat brain and spinal cord by electron microscopic autoradiography, Brain Res. 41:131, 1972.
National Drug and Therapeutic Index (Ambler, Pa., IMS America, July 1974–June 1975).
Rivera-Calimlim, L., Castaneda, L., and Lasagna, L.: Effects of mode of management on plasma chlorpromazine in psychiatric patients, Clin. Pharmacol. Ther. 14:978, 1973.
Saletu, B., Simeon, J., Saletu, M., et al.: Behavioral and visual evoked potential investigations during trihexyphenidyl and thiothixene treatment in psychotic boys, Biol. Psychiatry 8:177, 1974.
Schull, H. J., Wilkinson, G. R., Johnson, R., et al.: Normal disposition of oxazepam in acute hepatitis and cirrhosis, Ann. Intern. Med. 84:420, 1976.
Shader, R. I., and Greenblatt, D. J.: Clinical implications of benzodiazepines pharmacokinetics, Am. J. Psychiatry 134:652, 1977.
Shaw, C. R., Lockett, H. J., Lucas, A. R., et al.: Tranquilizer drugs in the treatment of emotionally disturbed children: I. Inpatients in a residential treatment center, J. Am. Acad. Child Psychiatry 2:725, 1963.
Stein, L., Wise, C. D., and Berger, B. D.: Antianxiety Action of Benzodiazepines: Decrease in Activity of Serotonin Neurons in the Punishment System, in Garattini, S. (ed): *The Benzodiazepines* (New York, Raven Press, 1973), pp. 299–326).
Takahashi, T., Konishi, S., Powell, D., et al.: Identification of the motor neuron-depolarizing peptide in bovine dorsal root as hypothalamic substance P, Brain Res. 73:59, 1974.

10/Drug Abuse and Drug Dependence

DRUG ABUSE in adolescents has increased dramatically during the last decade. It is not uncommon to find that 10–15% of American high school students are regular abusers of various substances. Drugs are also being pushed in junior high schools, where a fair number of students are experimenting with their use for the first time. Alcohol and marijuana appear to be the substances most abused by American youth.

The World Health Organization's Committee on Addiction-Producing Drugs proposes to replace the ambiguous and controversial terms "drug addiction" and "drug habituation" with "drug dependence." Drug dependence is defined as:

> a state arising from repeated administration of a drug on a periodic or continuous basis. Its characteristics will vary with the agent involved, and this must be made clear by designating the particular type of drug dependence in each specific case—for example, drug dependence of the morphine type, of cocaine type, of cannabis type, of barbiturate type, of amphetamine type, etc.

Drug Dependence

Marijuana

Among American youth, marijuana is the second most commonly abused substance after alcohol. Increasing numbers of teenagers in high school are smoking marijuana with a frequency varying from 1 to 3–4 times weekly. Most teenagers combine marijuana with alcohol on weekend parties or on outings, but roughly 1 marijuana user in 10 seems to be a daily smoker and will confine its use, typically, to nighttime. About 1–2% of all users are high during all their waking hours. Tetrahydrocannabinol (THC) is regarded as the major psychoactive ingredient in marijuana. Concentration of THC varies from 2 to 10% in grades and batches of marijuana. Marijuana is supplied on the streets either in leaf form or as a dried resin and are the types nearly always smoked in the United States. The leaf variety comes in the form of a loose, fine, dried herb (commonly called "grass"). It is sprinkled into cigarette papers and then rolled into a joint, a small, thin, marijuana cigarette. The resin form (commonly called "hashish") is usually smoked in a pipe. It normally comes to customers as a hard block that must be chipped or cut off in tiny pieces, which are then lit. The technique for smoking grass or hashish is the same. The smoker inhales deeply and holds the smoke in his lungs for as long as possible, then exhales slowly. The effects are felt within minutes of smoking high-quality marijuana, and within 10–15 minutes, the user is stoned. The effects last for several hours. Although the user is no longer under the influence of marijuana 4–6 hours after smoking it, traces of THC remain in the blood stream for about 72 hours.

It is almost impossible for a human being to overdose on marijuana. Although a great deal of psychological dependence is possible, no physical withdrawal symptoms occur during abstinence. Subjective experiences include decreased tension, relaxation, euphoria, increased hunger and a heightened sense of taste and hearing. There are few objective signs of marijuana smoking, except that the person may laugh easily and appear silly and giggly.

Barbiturates

Commonly used barbiturates are secobarbital (known as "sekkies" or "seggies" on the street), nembutal ("nemmies" or "nimbies"), or amytal and tuinal (a combination of amytal and secobarbital called "tooies"). The street names follow the colors and patterns of the capsules containing the drugs: rainbow, red bird, yellow jackets, reds.

An addict may take between 800 and 2,000 mg of barbiturates daily to satisfy his dependence. The time needed to produce dependence varies widely among different individuals. Moderately large doses can cause physical dependence within 4–6 weeks.

Barbiturate use has increased enormously among adolescents. It is not uncommon to see high school students stoned on "downers." Barbiturates and alcohol are similar in their effects, although not identical. The reflexes are diminished, coordination is impaired, feelings of anxiety and tension are reduced, sedation occurs, the speech is somewhat slurred, and the mind tends to be clouded. High doses induce sleep.

Narcotics

All narcotics are likely to produce addiction. Addictions have been found to occur with morphine, heroin, Dilaudid (dihydromorphinone), codeine and a few weaker preparations, such as paregoric, as well as synthetic narcotics, including meperidine (Demerol) and methadone (Dalophine). Heroin is probably the most potent of the narcotics by weight when pure, but it is almost never pure when purchased on the street. Heroin is currently an infrequently used narcotic among adolescents and young adults.

In the 1950s and 1960s, the use of heroin was almost exclusively confined to ghetto youth. Today, a much wider range of young people are trying and sometimes becoming addicted to heroin.

Withdrawal symptoms vary, depending on the strength of black market heroin and the frequency of use. A good deal of it is sufficiently potent to cause true physiologic addiction. Many addicts will escalate from a "nickel bag" (a packet costing $5.00) a day to 2, 3 or even 20 packets a day.

Patterns of heroin abuse differ widely. At one extreme, it is taken by intravenous injections (mainlining) several times a day with clock-like regularity. At the other extreme, it may be taken via the nasal route (snorting or sniffing) on a very irregular basis.

Medical pathologies (e.g., hepatitis, pneumonia) associated with street addiction (overdosing aside) do not result from the drug itself. Heavy, long-term addiction to narcotics, including heroin, does not damage or destroy human bodily tissue. In fact, ironically, in strictly organic terms, heroin is an extremely safe drug. The high mortality is caused not by the destructive action of heroin, but by overdosing and by secondary diseases commonly contracted by addicts.

The initial use of heroin is often extremely unpleasant. It is only after a number of administrations that the neophyte begins to enjoy its effects. Since the amount of heroin must be increased to maintain the same degree of pleasure, the typical life of a street junkie is dismal at best. A life of crime is almost inevitable in order to support the habit, which may cost from $15 to $100 or more a day. Many addicts talk of kicking the habit, but very few are able to do so on their own.

Stimulants

Mild stimulants, such as nicotine (cigarettes) and caffeine (coffee), are part of most Americans' daily intake. The use of such stimulant drugs as amphetamines has increased a great deal in the United States. There are two fairly distinct patterns of amphetamine use: small-to-moderate doses are taken in quasi-legitimate, although sometimes illegal, circumstances by individuals not defined by society as criminal or deviant, i.e., depressed persons, the harried businessman, the long-haul truckdriver, the ambitious athlete, the anxious student cramming for an exam. These individuals use amphetamines to attain a mental or physical state conducive to some practical end of which society approves. The amount consumed by such people usually ranges from 5 to 10 mg in single doses.

The second group consists of people who use large doses of amphetamines in order to become high. These abusers may consume from 100 mg to 1,000 mg or more a day.

Withdrawal of amphetamines rarely causes severe physical symptoms, other than insomnia.

Cocaine

Cocaine is rarely used in this country. It may be taken orally (as snuff) or intravenously. In moderate dosage, it causes nervousness, apprehension and trembling. Physical symptoms may include tachycardia, hypertension and mydriasis. Large dosages may produce a toxic psychosis, including auditory, visual and tactile hallucinations and delusions. Withdrawal can be accomplished easily, since it does not produce severe physical symptoms.

Glue Sniffing

Glue sniffing is very common in young teenagers. Excessive glue sniffing produces euphoria and excitement, followed by ataxia and slurred speech which may last 30–45 minutes. In some cases, drowsiness, stupor and coma may ensue. The practice is quite habituating for many children and may drive them to steal in order to satisfy their habit. However, there is no evidence of physiologic dependence.

Abstinence Syndrome in Adolescents

Most drug abusers who have become drug dependent are somehow able to find drugs to supply their needs, but some young adults, stranded in areas away from the sources of their drug supply, will show symptoms of withdrawal. From a therapeutic standpoint, it is important to be familiar with these symptoms while helping such a person with his dependence.

The most commonly abused drugs that give rise to severe withdrawal symptoms are alcohol, narcotics and barbiturates. Alcohol withdrawal is rarely seen in adolescents, but addiction to narcotics and barbiturates is fairly frequent in the high school age group. Amphetamines, cocaine, LSD and marijuana do not cause severe withdrawal symptoms.

Narcotics

Withdrawal symptoms from morphine and heroin appear within 12–14 hours of the last dose. The initial signs are yawning, rhinorrhea, lacrimation, sweating, piloerection, pupillary dilation and restlessness. Later, muscular aches and twitches, insomnia, hypertension, abdominal cramps, vomiting, diarrhea, anorexia, profuse sweating, agitation and weight loss develop. In addition, spontaneous ejaculation may occur in males and profuse menstrual bleeding may ensue in females. These withdrawal symptoms are at their peak intensity between 48 and 72 hours after the last dose, then diminish and are virtually gone by 7–10 days. However, the patient often continues to complain of sleep difficulties, myalgia, weakness and malaise for several weeks and of autonomic imbalance, as manifested by an abnormal cold pressor response which may persist for up to 6 months. If at any time during the abstinence period a single dose of morphine is administered, all the abstinence phenomena quickly subside, only to reappear within 4–6 hours.

Therapeutic withdrawal is initiated to allow the patient to lead a satisfying and useful life without medically unwarranted use of drugs. This is best carried out in a hospital setting, where supportive medical and psychological services are routinely available as part of the therapeutic milieu. A detailed history and thorough physical examination are essential in every case. Specific details are required about which drugs have been used, in what amounts and with what frequency. This information is particularly important in cases of barbiturate addiction, since sudden withdrawal from barbiturates may cause convulsions. Urine examination for the presence of various drugs may provide additional information.

Two methods of withdrawal are frequently employed: rapid reduction and methadone substitution.

Rapid Reduction

Initially, the patient is stabilized for 2 or 3 days on a dose and frequency of subcutaneous injections of morphine sufficient to prevent the symptoms of abstinence. The size of the dose and the frequency of injections are based on the previous schedule of drug use, but it is rarely necessary to give more than 30 mg subcutaneously every 6 hours. Generally, morphine can substitute adequately for any opium derivative, but some difficulties may be encountered in cases of meperidine dependence.

After the initial stabilization, reduction is made on a dose-to-dose basis, depending upon the health of the patient and the occurrence of withdrawal symptoms. The dosage is reduced daily, while keeping the 4 daily injections on the same schedule. When morphine has been reduced to 10 mg 4 times a day, codeine 30 mg, is administered with smaller amounts of morphine for 1 day, then codeine alone in decreasing dosage for 2 or 3 days. Other medications, such as aspirin for aches and pains and smaller amounts of barbiturates, may be prescribed for sleep. The patient is kept in the hospital for an additional 10 days after the last codeine dose. The need for additional rehabilitative and psychological services is determined during this period. A definite arrangement for these services is made before the patient is discharged.

Methadone Substitution

The patient is stabilized on methadone, given in aqueous solution orally twice a day. Generally, in abstinence, 1 mg of methadone can be considered equal to the suppressing potency of 3 or 4 mg of morphine or 1 mg of heroin. In cases of uncertainty as to the accustomed dosage of opioids, a first trial dose of 10 mg of methadone is given. Subsequent doses are adjusted on the basis of the patient's response. In most cases, 10 to 20 mg of methadone orally twice daily suffices.

After the initial stabilization, the methadone is reduced gradually over a period of 3–10 days. Further rehabilitation is carried out as described above in the rapid reduction method.

Barbiturates

The earliest signs of abstinence syndrome are insomnia, weakness, restlessness, sweating and shakiness, with feelings of anxiety and apprehension. Later, abdominal cramps, vomiting, pains all over the body, convulsions and sometimes coma may occur.

Initially, the patient is stabilized on the same amount of barbiturates that he has been taking. The dosage may, however, have to be increased if the patient becomes oversedated.

When a patient is unable to recall his total daily dosage, a test dose is recommended. The suggested test dose is 200 mg of pentobarbital by mouth. It is given (on an empty stomach) to a patient who does not appear to be sedated. Half that amount is given to debilitated and elderly patients, whose condition is evaluated 1 hour later. If the abstinence syndrome is still evident, the same dose is repeated. If the patient lacks tolerance to pentobarbital, he may be sound asleep but is arousable. If he is awake but somewhat somnolent and experiencing nystagmus, slurred speech and considerable ataxia, he is probably able to tolerate 500–600 mg of pentobarbital daily. If he shows only lateral nystagmus without ataxia or somnolence, he may tolerate as much as 800 mg daily. If he shows no signs of intoxication 1 hour after receiving 200 mg of pentobarbital, he can probably tolerate 1,000 to 1,200 mg or more daily.

After stabilization, the pentobarbital is reduced gradually, about 10% of the daily dose each day. The patient should be examined daily for signs of intoxication or withdrawal. If signs of abstinence appear, reduction is carried out more slowly. The patient should be kept in the hospital for 10–15 days after complete withdrawal, with rehabilitative and psychological services provided as necessary.

Barbiturates and Opioids

It is not uncommon for some addicts to simultaneously abuse both barbiturates and narcotics. In these cases, the patient is first stabilized on both morphine (or methadone) and barbiturates. Pentobarbital is given orally in doses that are just sufficient to produce symptoms of mild intoxication, i.e., nystagmus, mild ataxia and perhaps slight slurring of speech. Stabilization on barbiturates is continued while withdrawal of morphine or methadone substitution is completed. Only thereafter should a gradual reduction of pentobarbital be carried out (not exceeding 100 mg a day). Should minor abstinence symptoms appear, such as trembling, sweating, insomnia, anorexia or postural hypotension, further reduction of pentobarbital is suspended until the symptoms disappear. Complete withdrawal of pentobarbital may take a month or longer, depending upon the extent of habitual dosage and frequency.

Management of Drug Intoxication

Morbidity and mortality associated with the use of various addictive drugs were fairly high a decade ago. Programs of methadone substitution, widespread awareness of drug dependence in young people and familiarity with the treatment of drug intoxication have reduced the mortality despite the increase in the total number of drug abusers.

The most commonly encountered intoxications are produced by the ingestion of alcohol, narcotics, barbiturates, hallucinogens and amphetamines.

Intoxication with Narcotics

Patients who have overdosed with heroin or morphine classically present with pinpoint pupils (unless anorexia has caused dilation), areflexia, marked respiratory depression (from apnea to 2 or 3 shallow gasping breaths per minute) and a cyanotic, clammy pallor.

Treatment must be prompt to be effective, and proper measures are essential. The following recommendations are helpful in emergency therapy:

1. Establish an airway: Clean the patient's mouth. With the patient in the supine position, tip the head slightly back. Pull the tongue forward, making certain it is not occluding the posterior oropharynx. Breathe for

the patient if he is apneic. Endotracheal intubation is frequently necessary.

2. Quickly assess the cardiovascular system: External cardiac massage, defibrillation and pacing may be necessary if the heartbeat is absent. In severe cases of narcotic overdosage, the cardiovascular system may be so depressed that pulmonary edema develops, and intubation or tracheostomy plus continuous positive pressure respiration may be life-saving.

3. Continue treatment for heroin or morphine overdosage as follows: *(a)* give 1 cc (1 cc/mg) levallorphan tartrate (Lorfan) or 1 cc (1 cc/5 mg) N-allylnonmorphine hydrochloride (Nalline) intravenously. These drugs take effect in seconds when given intravenously, while intramuscular injection may take 20 minutes or more. If the patient has collapsed veins, as many addicts do, try the external jugular or the femoral veins. *(b)* Give 3 to 5 cc (1 cc/20 mg) doxapram hydrochloride (Dopram) intravenously. This is a safe, temporary (lasting 3–5 minutes), nonspecific respiratory stimulant. However, it usually produces an immediate effect; thus an open airway should be ensured beforehand. *(c)* If the patient fails to respond, follow established emergency procedures to secure a route for administering intravenous fluids—preferably, with a large cannula. If moderate to severe acidosis is suspected, administer sodium bicarbonate. Begin the administration of a glucose-electrolyte solution. Draw blood for chemistries. Search for other etiology, such as evidence of trauma, blood loss, acute infectious process or increased intracranial pressure. *(d)* If long-standing drug depression is suspected, hospitalization, vigorous pulmonary therapy and aggressive antibiotic therapy are indicated.

Barbiturate Intoxication

Acute barbiturate intoxication is a fatal form of poisoning in which the eventual clinical outcome is often solely related to the level of supervision and care that is provided by attending physicians and nurses.

An elemental knowledge of the clinical pharmacology of barbiturates is an absolute prerequisite to optimum and intelligent management. The duration of action of any barbiturate is determined by a complex interaction among many variables: dose, rate of absorption, rate of metabolic degradation or excretion of the active drug, drug tolerance and rate of removal of nonmetabolized and active drug from the central nervous system. There is a good correlation between the duration of action and the mechanism by which the active drug is eliminated from the body. Short-acting agents (pentobarbital, secobarbital) are principally eliminated via hepatic degradation, with subsequent excretion of inactive metabolites in the urine. Hepatic degradation plays a lesser role in the elimination of long- and intermediate-acting agents (e.g., phenobarbital, amobarbital). The renal excretion of an unaltered and, therefore, active drug provides a much more important route of disposal for these agents.

Acute barbiturate intoxication must always be differentiated from other forms of coma or central nervous system injury. The depth of coma is often greater than might be expected from the plasma barbiturate concentration alone if alcohol and barbiturate ingestion have occurred concomitantly. Patients with barbiturate intoxication usually arrive in shock and coma. Corneal and deep tendon reflexes are absent, and pupillary response to light is minimal. Rectal temperature may be reduced to 95F. The skin of the ear lobes, nose or fingers is often cyanotic, reflecting the marked impairment in ventilation, there may be a modest increase in heart rate, the systolic blood pressure is generally reduced to 80 mm Hg and rhonchi and rales may be present on chest examination.

Initial physical examination should include an assessment of the vital signs, the extent of respiratory depression, the depth of coma and a search for evidence of trauma and neurologic abnormalities. Evidence of preexisting disease, such as hypertension, cirrhosis and diabetes mellitus, must be sought. The odor of the breath may indicate the presence of associated alcohol ingestion or diabetic ketoacidosis. Special attention should be paid to the status of corneal and deep tendon reflexes, the pupillary light reflex, bowel sounds and the response to verbal commands and deep painful stimuli.

Minimal laboratory evaluation at the time of first examination should incude roentgenographic examination of the chest and skull, routine urinalysis and estimates of hematocrit, WBC and differential counts. Blood should be obtained for typing and cross-matching, and an aliquot should be saved for future drug analysis if necessary. When available, measurements of blood urea nitrogen concentration, pH, plasma concentration of electrolytes, total barbiturates and creatinine should be obtained.

Regardless of the exact diagnosis, treatment should be instituted immediately if acute barbiturate intoxication is suspected. Management of circulatory and respiratory collapse represents an immediate therapeutic problem (which is handled in the manner described under narcotic intoxication).

Caloric intake must be maintained with parenteral fluids. Water and electrolyte losses must be replaced, and any site of infection must be detected and treated promptly. The eyes may be patched to prevent corneal damage. The patient should be placed on an alternative pressure type mattress, which is turned frequently. Good hygiene must be observed.

Other procedures, such as gastric saline lavage with activated charcoal, use of analeptic drugs, such as amphetamine, ethamivan (Emivan), diuretics, hemodialysis or peritoneal dialysis, should be considered in each case if deterioration continues.

The overall mortality is generally less than 5–7%, but follow-up care and rehabilitation of these addicts is extremely important.

Amphetamine Intoxication

Severe mental as well as physical symptoms may result from amphetamine intoxication. Mild symptoms of intoxication frequently occur in abusers of moderate amounts of amphetamine. The symptoms include restlessness, tremor, insomnia, talkativeness, irritability, dilation of pupils and sweating. Heavy users of amphetamine may suffer from confusion, delirium, hallucination, tachycardia, hypertension and may occasionally develop convulsions, cardiovascular collapse and coma.

Several drugs, such as chloroform, chloral hydrate, trisomoethanol, carbon tetrachloride or ethyl chloride, should be used with caution in association with amphetamines (especially epinephrine), since chloride, bromide and bromine derivatives of methane sensitize heart muscle to epinephrine and predispose to ventricular fibrillation.

Treatment of intoxication caused by this general group should consist of delaying the absorption of the ingested drug by giving tap water or milk and charcoal, then removing them by gastric lavage or emetics, followed by saline catharsis.

Specific treatment consists of the administration of central nervous system depressants, especially paraldehyde or a barbiturate. If convulsions appear imminent, a short-acting barbiturate should be given intravenously. Chlorpromazine, 1–2 mg/kg given intramuscularly, is very effective in controlling marked central nervous system excitation and concomitant hypertension. It may be repeated as necessary. If cardiovascular collapse occurs, blood pressure should be maintained with levarterenol and O_2, and artificial respiration should be given for shallow respiration or cyanosis. Ample fluid intake must be maintained, since the kidneys are the major route of excretion.

Intoxication with Hallucinogens

Hallucinogens are defined as substances that, administered in pharmacologic doses, create gross distortions in perception without significantly disturbing consciousness. In addition to producing frequent hallucinations, these substances exert a profound influence on mood, thought and behavior. The symptoms resemble the disturbances seen in naturally occurring psychoses.

There are four major chemical classes of hallucinogens: the indol alkaloid derivatives, the piperidine derivatives, the phenylethylamines and the cannabinols. The most commonly abused hallucinogens are lysergic acid diethylamide (LSD), amphetamine and marijuana. Amphetamine and marijuana do not produce hallucinations in pharmacologic doses and perhaps are not properly classified here. LSD is, however, a potent psychotogenic drug.

LSD is more than 8,000 times more potent on a dosage basis than mescaline. Less than 0.3 gm of LSD has caused the death of a 7,000 pound elephant in status epilepticus. It is effective at a dosage as low as 1 mg/kg of body weight in man. Thirty milligrams given by mouth produces various autonomic and psychological effects. During the first 4½ hours after ingestion, there is a clear-cut self-recognition of the drug's effect, followed by another 4–5 hour period in which the subjective sense of change is less marked, and there is a heightened self-centeredness and ideas of reference. At 12–24 hours after ingestion, there may be some letdown and slight fatigue. Psychological changes occur in mainly 3 areas: bodily sensation, affect and perception. Bodily sensations are characterized by a split of the self into two—one self being a relatively passive monitor observing a second self, which receives vivid experiences and perceptions. A dominant experience of self observing self can be experienced in a variety of ways—mystical, aesthetic or religious. There is an altered relationship of the body to its surroundings. One may perceive one's body fused to other objects or persons in the surroundings, and the sense of gravity may be distorted.

Perceptual qualities gain a life of their own, e.g., redness may become more interesting than the object that is red, or, more abstractly, "meaningfulness" may become more important than what is really meant. Distortions of shape and proportion are frequent.

Several contrary feelings may coexist. Since it is usually difficult to focus on one feeling, the subject fluctuates between laughing and crying, especially during the first 4 hours after drug ingestion.

Changes in the autonomic system may include tachycardia, mydriasis, rise in body temperature and hyperglycemia.

There are usually 3 broad categories of symptoms for which an LSD user may seek medical help: panic state, flashbacks and acute psychosis. Panic is more likely to occur in a novice than in an experienced user. Panic results from the user's inability to handle visual and auditory hallucinations and other perceptual distortions. It is usually the fear of losing one's control that precipitates panic. About half of these panic-striken patients can be successfully treated in the emergency room with intramuscular injection of chlorpromazine (Thorazine). These patients may be discharged in a few hours. Patients who remain in a panic state in spite of assurances and tranquilizers require hospitalization. The following principles of treatment should be kept in mind while managing these persons:

1. Reduce environmental stimulation and provide a quiet room.
2. Reduce the strangeness of the environment—ask somebody from home or a close friend to stay with the patient. Provide less frequent changes of nurses.
3. Reassure the patient that he will recover—relaxation and serenity are mandatory.
4. Administer tranquilizers, such as Thorazine, chlordiazepoxide (Librium) or Valium liberally.
5. After recovery, provide a retrospective interpretation of the delusional and hallucinatory experiences.

Recovery is generally rapid and occurs within 3 days in most cases.

The second reason for LSD users' seeking medical help is the occurrence of flashbacks. Flashbacks are reappearances of sensory and visual experiences in the absence of recent LSD ingestion. The perceptual distortions associated with feelings of depersonalization may cause fright and occasional panic. These effects are reported to have occurred up to one year after the last ingestion of the drug. Unless the user is panic-stricken, he is usually treated on an outpatient basis. Moderately large doses of phenothiazines, such as Thorazine, may be necessary to control the flashbacks.

Occurrence of acute psychosis, although somewhat uncommon, is generally a grave situation. The psychotic reaction may last a few weeks or may continue for years in some cases. It is possible to distinguish between a panic reaction and an acute psychotic reaction from LSD by the ability of the person to recognize his experiences as foreign. A person in panic describes his experiences as unusual and recognizes his inability to control them. A person in acute psychosis loses this critical judgment, believes his perceptual distortions to be real and allows his behavior to be guided by the nature of the distortions.

Abstinence Syndrome in the Newborn

The first description of a neonatal narcotic withdrawal syndrome appeared in the medical literature almost a century ago. Many articles have been published since that time, most of them during the past two decades. Early recognition and therapy of affected infants have been shown to result in prompt control of symptoms and a good prognosis for survival.

Morphine and its derivatives, as well as a number of other abused drugs, have been known to cross the placenta. Analysis of the blood, tissues and urine of newborn infants has confirmed the presence of morphine, meperidine, methadone, barbiturates and other drugs taken before delivery.

Drugs which cross the placenta may exert two types of effects on the fetus: those which are unique to the particular developmental stage of the fetus at the time of exposure and those which can be predicted on the basis of effects observed in adults. Little is known about effects of the first type. Effects of the second type are exemplified as the "neonatal narcotic withdrawal syndrome."

The infant who has been chronically exposed to narcotics taken by his mother during pregnancy is suddenly deprived of his source of drugs at the time of delivery. If he has developed physiologic dependence, abstinence symptoms may be expected to ensue. Symptoms, if they occur, are usually seen in both mother and infant, unless they are modified by a continued intake of narcotic drugs or by other medication. However, some infants may become symptomatic, while their mothers remain symptom-free, or, more rarely, an infant may remain asymptomatic, while his mother develops withdrawal symptoms. The infant whose mother has been drug-free for a week or more prior to delivery generally does not show signs of withdrawal syndrome.

Withdrawal symptoms usually begin during the first 24 hours after birth. Occasionally, symptoms may be observed at birth or are delayed for as long as 4 days. The more gradual onset in some infants is perhaps related to a short interval between the mother's last dose and delivery, to the effect of medications administered during labor and to relatively slower metabolism and excretion by the immature infant.

The cardinal symptoms of neonatal narcotic withdrawal syndrome are coarse tremors, hyperactivity, irritability and a number of other symptoms, including vomiting, poor feeding, increased muscle tone, nasal stuffiness, sneezing, yawning, skin abrasions secondary to excessive activity, persistent, angry crying, sweating and loose stools. Tachycardia with respiratory alkalosis may also be associated with the syndrome.

Severe diarrhea is unusual in the absence of other causes, such as enteric infection. Severe tremors or myoclonic jerks may sometimes be misinterpreted as seizures. True convulsions should always raise the suspicion of another etiology, such as hypoglycemia, hypocalcemia, meningitis or withdrawal from drugs other than narcotics. Abrupt withdrawal of barbiturates, alcohol or some tranquilizers may precipitate convulsions.

Diagnosis of neonatal narcotic withdrawal syndrome is not difficult when the history of maternal drug abuse is known and characteristic signs are observed in the infant. In the case of denial, physical examination of the mother for stigmata, such as needle marks and thrombostic veins, or withdrawal signs may reveal the source of the infant's difficulties.

Symptoms of narcotic withdrawal may subside within a week or may persist for as long as several weeks. Observations suggest a relatively short period of disturbed behavior manifested by sleeplessness and crying for 2–3 months, hyperphagia, hyperacusis and outbursts of screaming for as long as 6 months.

The syndrome is self-limiting and, in milder cases, subsides in a few days with no specific therapy. A quiet, warm environment, gentle handling, swaddling and frequent small feedings are helpful, as are measures to minimize skin abrasions, such as placing the infant on a sheepskin or in a diaper hammock tied in his crib. Prophylactic therapy based solely upon a history of maternal drug intake would result in unnecessary treatment of many infants who remain asymptomatic or whose symptoms respond to simple supportive measures. No harm is done by a period of observation to determine the need for active treatment.

The most widely used drugs in the treatment of neonatal narcotic withdrawal syndrome have been paregoric (1–3 drops/kg every 3–6 hours), phenobarbital (8–10 mg/kg/24 hours in 4 divided doses) and chlorpromazine (2.5–4.5 mg/kg/24 hours in 4 divided doses). Most infants can be satisfactorily managed with a short course of less than a week of drug therapy. Medications should be discontinued or reduced after a few days and the infant observed. In many infants, acute withdrawal symptoms will not recur or, if they do, will be mild enough to be managed with only gentle handling and careful feeding. Original doses of medication should be resumed in cases of recurrence of moderate to severe symptoms, then gradually reduced over a period of a week or more.

Definite attention should be paid to rehabilitation of the mother before the infant is sent home with her.

Amphetamine and Cocaine

Abrupt discontinuance of prolonged use of amphetamine in adults leads to lethargy and psychological depression but not to a true abstinence syndrome. Most infants born to amphetamine users are symptom-free. Similarly, cocaine use does not produce true addiction and would not be expected to cause an abstinence syndrome in newborn infants.

Hallucinogens

There have been a number of reports of chromosomal damage and malformation of infants of mothers who were users of lysergic acid diethylamide (LSD). Although the relationship is far from conclusive, the available reports are sufficient to maintain a suspicion of LSD as a possible teratogenic substance.

It is reasonable to presume that the infant of a mother who delivered while under the influence of LSD might show some form of altered behavior. It is not known whether in utero exposure to LSD has an adverse effect on future neurologic, personality or intellectual development.

Studies of the teratogenic potential of marijuana are sparse, and little is known of the effect, if any, on the human fetus.

Barbiturates

Withdrawal symptoms in infants born to mothers who have been taking barbiturates closely resemble those seen in infants born to heroin addicts, except that they usually have a later onset. Symptoms generally develop between the 6th and 14th days of life. The delay may be the result of slower metabolism and slower excretion of barbiturates in newborns. The diagnosis of abstinence syndrome may be easily overlooked in infants whose symptoms do not develop until after routine discharge from the hospital nursery.

Minor Tranquilizers and Alcohol

Chronic use of minor tranquilizers and alcohol is known to produce an abstinence syndrome of the barbiturate type, with a similar risk of seizures and occasional fatalities.

Alcohol withdrawal manifested by tremor, irritability and sleepiness has been reported in some infants born to alcoholic mothers. It is probable that some infants born to mothers who have been chronic users of minor tranquilizers may develop an abstinence syndrome.

Methadone

Reduction of methadone dosage in late pregnancy in narcotic-addicted women is reported to reduce the incidence of neonatal narcotic withdrawal syndrome. Any reduction in methadone dosage, however, must be carefully monitored. Serial amniotic fluid catecholamine assay may be useful in monitoring infant stress during reduction of methadone dosage.

11/Management of Rape Victims

RAPE IS A crisis situation for most children and adolescents. Besides being overwhelmed with an excessive amount of aggression, the rape victim is very uncertain about the future consequences of the incident. Its legal and social implications defy the immediate comprehension of the young victims. Anxiety over pregnancy, disease, changed relationships with peers and parental rejection may be so extreme that it temporarily surpasses the shock of having been assaulted. These considerations make it mandatory to employ both medical and psychological services to reduce the intensity of anxiety, to mollify feelings of shame, guilt and self-incrimination and to help the victim to cope better with this traumatic situation. Failure to deal with guilt may result in profound depression in and self-incrimination by rape victims.

Statistics

Rape is statistically associated with other sorts of criminal activity. A rise in the incidence of rape is normally paralleled by increases in the incidence of murder, robbery and assault. In 1968, there were an estimated 31,060 attempted and statutory forceable rapes in the United States, an increase of 84% since 1960. In 1973, there were 51,000 reported cases, a staggering 60% rise over 1968. It is estimated that there is a 10–15% yearly rise in the incidence of rape in the United States, leading to a projection of about 85,000–90,000 reported cases by 1980.

Some of the rise may be attributed to the greater willingness of women to report the crime, but many victims are still hesitant to expose themselves to the ordeal of a trial. Various investigators have concluded that the reported figures are only a fraction of the actual incidence.

Large numbers of rape victims are females in their late teens and early 20s. About one fifth of all rape victims are young children under 13 years of age. The age of boy victims peaks at both 10 and 14 years, while the age for girl victims is relatively equally distributed throughout the early teen years with a slight rise at ages 10 and 12. The percentage of boy victims is very small (6–10%) and usually involves some kind of homosexual experience with peers of approximately the same age.

Black and poor women are overrepresented among the victims. Approximately one third to one half of the offenders are known by the child victims, while about one fourth of the offenders are known to the victims in their late teens or early 20s. Only about 15% of the offenders who are tried in court are convicted.

Emergency Room Hospital Visits by Rape Victims

Emergency room visits by a rape victim may be motivated by medical, legal and/or psychological needs. A large number of victims come in for an assessment of physical injuries, for a check-up for venereal disease and pregnancy and to receive treatment for wounds, lacerations and fractures. Some of the victims contact the police first and then come to a medical facility, either on their own or on instructions from the police. There are some victims who turn to a medical facility because they are simply overwhelmed, shocked, frightened and lonely and want to verbalize their terror.

Adolescent victims often try to give the appearance of being less worried and less stunned than they actually are, in their attempt to conceal the sexual nature of the assault. Many parents refuse vaginal examination because the adolescents involved have convinced them that they were only beaten up and not sexually assaulted. The parents of child and adolescent rape victims usually appear angry and helpless. It is not uncommon to see an enraged parent of a child victim pacing restlessly in the hospital emergency area and involuntarily communicating this rage to various hospital personnel. These parents require special handling. A hospital social worker is probably the best person to help these parents ventilate their feelings. They usually have many questions but are unable to ask the busy physician. Their questions relate to various legal, social and emotional problems. They wonder how they should explain the act to the young child, how they should react to her, and about the emotional consequences to the child's development and later sexual adjustment.

Taking the History

The history should be obtained by the physician in a private room in the presence of the parents. The child should also be interviewed alone to obtain some of the personal details which she may have withheld in the presence of her parents. The history should include the circumstances of the rape, a description of the assailant, the nature of the conversation between the assailant and the victim before and after the rape, threats of injury, whether there was a struggle, details of the physical and sexual assault, the history of such assaults and whether the victim has ever had venereal disease or been pregnant. The patient's feelings and worries about the incident may be explored more fully during individual interviews.

Although efforts should also be made to explore the past emotional and social difficulties of the child and the child-parent relationship, reliable information on this topic is frequently impossible to obtain because of the heightened emotional situation surrounding the trauma. This portion of the history may thus be best deferred until follow-up interviews.

Physical Examination

Physical examination should include the general appearance of the patient, condition of the clothes, smell of urine and semen from the clothes, detailed notation of bruises, lacerations and bleeding, x-ray of suspected fractures and an assessment of internal bleeding.

Permission is required for vaginal examination, which should be performed in the presence of a nurse or female police officer. The vaginal examination of a young child who is crying and bleeding profusely may require general anesthesia. In the absence of any noticeable general injury, the vaginal examination may be avoided in most young children, since it is not necessary for the prosecution of the case. A hasty vaginal examination of a young child under highly emotionally charged circumstances following an alleged rape can only exacerbate psychological trauma and may be of little medical or legal value. One must decide if there are clear indications for vaginal examination beforehand: lacerations or bruises in the genital area certainly require further exploration.

A senior pediatric or gynecology resident should perform the vaginal examination, if possible. The primary objective is to ascertain whether the incident occurred as alleged by the victim. Entrance of the penis within the labia minora may be sufficient to establish rape. Evidence of use of force by the assailant should also be sought. The information derived from the vaginal examination may frequently be limited, and one must be extremely conservative in drawing conclusions from anything but frankly visible traumatic conditions, such as a bruised or bleeding vulva or a freshly and characteristically traumatized hymen.

Pubic hair should be combed, and all the collected hair should be submitted as a separate specimen for laboratory evaluation to differentiate between male and female hair. Two sets of swabs or aspirated fluids from the vagina should be collected, one for the legal authorities and one for the hospital. The specimens are examined for sperm by a wet smear, and a gram stain for *Neisseria gonorrhoeae* is done for further identification of organisms. A quantitative determination of acid phosphatase is also carried out for semen. A repeat serology and pregnancy test is advised after 6 weeks.

The report should be written in two parts: the first part should describe the factual findings from the physical examination, the second part may include one's conclusions and impressions with regard to the occurrence of rape, degree of violence, degree of struggle and resistance, and, if possible, the psychological status of the patient. The following protocol (suggested by Hunter, 1977) may be used as a quick checklist for appraisal and management of rape victims:

I. Initial observation before examination
   - Mental state:
   - Physical state:
     - Clothing:
     - Dirt:
     - Debris:

II. History
   - History of incident:
     - Where contacted:
     - Circumstances of the rape:
     - What happened afterward:
   - Specific questions:
     - Any physical violence?
     - Any threats?
     - Any weapons seen or alluded to?
     - Has the patient cleaned up or bathed or douched since the episode?
     - Condom on assailant?
     - Douche used before the episode?
   - Ob/Gyn history:
     - History of serious illnesses, including venereal disease:
     - Date of last menstrual period:
     - Pregnancy protection, if any:
     - Date of last prior sexual intercourse:

III. Physical examination (the patient's entire body should be scanned for injuries. Note the approximate age of the injuries).
   - Superficial examination:
     - Cuts:
     - Scrapes:
     - Bruises:
     - Debris:
   - Pelvic examination:
     - Debris:

Lacerations:
Bleeding:
Introitus:
Vagina:
Cervix:
Uterus:
Adnexa:

IV. Laboratory cultures to be obtained (all slides should be labeled by the physician or by the nurse in the physician's presence).
__Two dry slides, air dried
__One slide preserved in ethyl alcohol bottle
__One wet mount to be checked by the examining doctor
__Transgrow culture medium
__Vaginal vault wash: 10 cc sterile saline, placed in rubber-top blood container tube
__VDRL
Laboratory tests placed in refrigerator by ______________

V. Other considerations (The patient should be prophylactically treated for venereal disease).
Drugs used and dosage:
Prophylaxis for pregnancy prevention; pregnancy test:
Any torn or bloody clothing is considered evidence and should be saved until released by the police
__Follow-up arranged
With whom? ________________________________

Examination of the Offender

Occasionally the offender is apprehended immediately and is also brought for physical examination. The accused may be examined only with his written consent. The man has the legal right not to give any history and should be made aware of this right before being asked for any details. Physical examination under court order obviates prior consent.

The physical examination should include a general survey of the man's appearance and clothing. Any damp patches should be noted, and the appropriate parts of the clothing removed for laboratory examination. Presence and location of scratches, bruises, reddening of knees, blood stains and traces of lipstick should be noted. The genital organs may show evidence of recent emission of semen, bruises and scratches. A sample of pubic hair is collected by combing. Also gathered are hair on other parts of the body or clothes. A blood sample is taken for grouping. Blood stains on the body or on clothes are collected separately for grouping.

A report should be prepared along the same lines as suggested for examination of the victim.

Treatment of the Victim

An ideal treatment plan includes immediate medical services for the victim, psychological support for the patient as well as for the parents and legal advice and follow-up medical or psychological services as needed.

Immediate Medical Treatment

In addition to the treatment of bodily injuries, prophylactic treatment for venereal disease is commonly administered in all suspected rape cases. A single intramuscular injection of 2,400,000 units of benzadine penicillin G is sufficient. In the presence of penicillin allergy, 500 mg of tetracycline 4 times/day for 15 days is adequate. A 5-day regimen of diethylstilbestrol 25 mg 2 times/day to prevent possible pregnancy is offered to the patient if she is not already pregnant or is inadequately protected with contraceptives. Diethylstilbestrol may cause a great deal of nausea and occasional mesonephric adenocarcinoma of the vagina in female offspring if used during the first trimester of gestation. Conjugated equine estrogenic substances, 2.5 mg tabs given 4 times daily for 5 days, are equally effective and produce less nausea and risk of malignancy. The patient should be told that such drug protection is not guaranteed to be completely effective. If menstruation does not ensue within a week after cessation of estrogen therapy, dilatation and curettage should be considered.

Immediate Psychological Support

Immediate psychological support is best provided by an experienced hospital social worker, who should be called to the emergency room in all cases of rape. The parents usually have much to ventilate and have many questions to ask. The worker may not be able to answer all their questions, especially those related to the effect of rape on the emotional development of the child. The parents should be told that different children react differently to rape and that the worker needs to know more about the child before answering such questions. The generalization that most children do quite well is usually not very helpful. The initial session can best be used to build up a supportive relationship and provide guidance with regard to the medical and legal procedures.

Follow-Up

Follow-up services consist primarily of psychological counseling, which should be carried out, if possible, by the same social worker who initially talked with the parents. These follow-up visits provide a better opportunity for exploration of the social and emotional adjustment of the child, parental attitude toward the child and the family's reaction to the incident. Different parents react differently: some become overprotective and impose unnecessary restrictions on the child, while others may blame and ridicule their daughter for having been raped. Sometimes, the incident brings marital conflicts out into the open. The parents fight and argue, using their differences of opinion over the management of the child as the starting point.

Young children generally do not contribute much during follow-up visits. In some cases, frequent play therapy sessions may be necessary to bring out the child's anxiety and other conflicts related to the rape. Other children and adolescents become more verbal about their experience and frequently adjust better if the parents are accepting and nonpunitive. A few children develop severe phobic reactions to going outside or to school. These are serious psychological consequences and require immediate psychiatric treatment.

Some families feel extremely ashamed of the incident and avoid any follow-up visits. Telephone contacts have been fairly successful with these families, who are often quite willing to converse on the telephone but want to avoid clinic visits.

Several clinics keep a list of older adolescents or adults who have been raped in the past and are willing to share their experiences with the new rape victim. These people, however, should be screened carefully with regard to their emotional adjustment before they are put on such a list. Talking to such a person, even by telephone, may at times be extremely supportive to the recent rape victim.

Legal Aspects

Rape may be defined as "unlawful carnal knowledge of a woman by force." Three elements are necesssary to constitute rape: carnal knowledge, force and commission of the act without consent. The slightest penetration of the male organ is sufficient to constitute carnal knowledge. Emission of semen is not necessary. Penetration must be proved beyond a reasonable doubt, but circumstantial evidence may be sufficient. Force may be defined as "actual physical force or coercion by threats or intimidation." In all states, females below a specified age (which varies from 14 to 18 years) are presumed incapable of consent. Intercourse with a woman below this stated age is legally defined as statutory rape. In addition, a woman under the influence of alcohol or drugs to the point that she does not know what she is doing is legally considered incapable of giving consent.

Effects on Later Adjustment

Freud's earlier papers (1896) hypothesized that the cause of hysteria was a passive sexual experience (or traumatic seduction) before puberty. This hypothesis was later modified so that actual seduction was not necessary. Fantasied seduction could have the same result, since in the child's mind truth is not distinguishable from emotional fiction. Freud repeatedly emphasized the importance of infantile sexual life to subsequent sexual development. He believed that very few children would escape some kind of sexual activity or sexual experience before puberty: "It is my conviction that no child—none at least who is mentally sound, still less one who is mentally gifted—can avoid being occupied with sexual problems in the years before puberty" (1908). He concluded that actual seduction might hasten and stimulate the sexual development of the child.

Melanie Klein (1932) believed sexual relations in childhood were a frequent occurrence. Such sexual relationships might, she believed, have a less detrimental influence in later life if they occurred with a helping and loving person, such as a brother, cousin or friend. Klein also believed that an overly sadistic partner arouses more anxiety and guilt and anger toward men and thus would have a more detrimental effect on later sexual adjustment.

Ferenczi (1933) stressed:

> The most important change produced in the mind of the child by the anxiety, fear-ridden identification with the adult partner, is the introduction of the guilt feelings of the adults, which make hitherto harmless play appear as a punishable offence. . . . When the child recovers from such an attack, it feels enormously confused, in fact, split—innocent and culpable at the same time and its confidence in the testimony of its sense is broken. . . . The playful trespasses of the child are raised to serious reality only by the passionate, often infuriated, punitive sanctions and lead to depressive states in the child, who until then felt blissfully guiltless.[1]

Rabinovitch (1953) stated that early sexual contact with adults led to the

---

[1]Ferenczi: *Psychoanal. Q.* 2:361, 1933.

development of a compulsive need to reexperience gratification at a genital level and to an acting-out type of sexual delinquency in adolescence.

In a follow-up study of 60 children who had been sexually assaulted by adults, Moses (1932) found that 8 years after the incident well over half of the victims had difficulties in emotional adjustment.

In another follow-up study of 54 children, aged 9–13 years, selected from court files, Augusta Rasmussen (1934) found that 20–30 years after the rape incident, all but 8 subjects were well adjusted. The author felt that the poor adjustment of the 8 patients was not attributable to the sexual assault.

Bender and Grugett (1952) followed a group of 14 children who had received an extensive psychiatric evaluation at the time of their admission to the hospital soon after the rape incident. Fifteen years later, they found that 9 of the children had adjusted satisfactorily, 1 (who had been seduced by a parent) had become psychotic and 4 (who were intellectually deficient) had achieved little personal adjustment.

Landis (1956) administered a questionnaire which included questions on family background, maturation and sexual experiences to a group of 1,800 college students. Thirty percent of the men and 35% of the women reported at least one experience with a sexual deviate. The author concluded that, in general, the great majority of the victims seemed to have recovered rather soon without acquiring a permanently conflicting attitude toward sex from the experience. Only 2.2% of the women with deviate experience and 0.4% of the men felt that they had gained undesirable ideas about sex from their experience. Sexual experiences with family members were found to be more traumatic than sexual experiences with a rapist.

Sometimes the reaction of the parents or the police may disturb the child more seriously than the sexual contact itself. Preoccupation with the incident is generally abandoned if the social consequences of the assault are minimal and the child is provided with an accepting home and school environment.

Not all sexual assaults on children by adults lead to subsequent personality problems. Brutal and sadistic assaults, however, are likely to arouse a great deal of fear, anxiety and sometimes guilt in relation to subsequent sexual acts. Such sexual assaults may also cause an increase in autoerotic habits. In some children, early seduction may lead to a pattern of sexual acting-out.

Personality Dynamics of Victims

Kinsey reported (1953) that 24% of the females in his sample had preadolescent sexual contacts with adult males. The highest frequency of contacts occurred in the poor sections of the city. Most children were between 10 and 12 years of age at the time of approach. They were exposed mostly to exhibitionism, fondling and manipulation of genitalia. Only 3% of the children were involved in actual coitus. The majority of the children (80%) had been involved in only one incident, and the remaining 20% had taken part in several incidents.

Some seductions are actively desired by children and are frequently attributed to difficulties in the parent-child relationship. Johnson (1953) believed that in every case in which the child was a willing participant, one or both parents had serious problems at the genital level. One or both parents unconsciously sanctioned or fostered the child's acting-out of the parents' poorly integrated, forbidden impulses. As the parents achieved vicarious gratification of these impulses, they often at the same time expressed the hostility inherent in their conflicts in a destructive fashion toward the child.

Eissler (1950) felt that mothers defended themselves from their own guilt feelings for these impulses by using the child as a scapegoat.

Blos (1961) described two different patterns of development of sexual delinquency that he attributed to parental inadequacy. In the first type, the girl becomes aware of her father's inadequacy from observation of her mother's dissatisfaction with the father and turns to sexual acting-out to possess an ideal oedipal object and to punish her mother for rejecting her father. In the second type, regression to preoedipal passivity occurs due to the difficult oedipal situation, such as the inadequacy of the father. Wild expression of heterosexuality is used as a defense against the oral dependency needs of these youngsters.

Weiss et al. (1955) emphasized the dichotomy between accidental and participating rape victims. Of 73 girls studied, 21 were thought to be accidental victims and 44 to have participated in the affair. In the remaining 8 cases, no decision about involvement could be reached. Participating victims were attractive girls who frequently had more than one sexual experience with an adult, who was often a friend of the victim. The relationship was kept secret from the parents until it was discovered. Accidental victims, by contrast, were usually younger, had no previous sexual experience, did not know the offender and told the parents promptly of the incident. The study indicated that the sexual acting-out by the participating victims was not free from remorse and guilt. These girls had many phobias, nightmares and anxieties. They were also inclined to be sexually promiscuous, had been truant from school, had run away from home and manifested extreme fluctuations of mood.

Several studies have found that a fairly large proportion of rape victims are in the low-average or borderline range of intelligence. In a study of 98 sexually abused children, Lafon et al. (1958) found that 49% had an I.Q. of less than 70. Burton (1968) studied a group of sexually assaulted children along with several control groups matched for age, sex, I.Q., class attainment, religion and socioeconomic status. Adjustment in school was measured by the Bristol Social Adjustment Guides, filled in by classroom teachers. Personality structure was assessed by Thematic Apperception Test (TAT) stories. Burton concluded that there was no evidence in the TAT themes of an excessive anxiety or fear of violence or injury. He noticed, however, a tendency toward "unsettledness and unforthcomingness" more frequently in children whose assault had taken place only a short while before the test. This tendency diminished in severity with time. There was a significant difference in affection-seeking behavior between assaulted children and those in the control groups.

Personality Dynamics of Offenders

Seghorn (1971) differentiated 33 convicted rapists into three groups on the basis of their responses to a battery of psychological tests. In the first group, the act of rape represented displaced aggression from other frustrating situations. The sexual behavior was used in the service of the primary, aggressive aim to physically harm the victim. In the second group, an unconsummated and ineffectual rape attempt was made simply to establish an adult heterosexual relationship. The third group consisted of impulsive rapists who closely fitted the classic formulation of psychopath or impulsive character disorder. The rape appeared to be but a sexual manifestation of the general inability to delay gratification. Seghorn concluded that there was no one unvarying set of personality dynamics underlying the behavior of the sex offender. The sex offense resulted from various types of conflict and personality problems.

Perdue and Lester (1972) compared the Rorschach responses of 15 convicted rapists with 15 men convicted of aggressive, nonsexual crimes. They concluded that the rapists did not differ from those convicted of aggressive, nonsexual crimes.

Several studies have investigated the effects of obscenity and pornography in promoting sex offenses. Gebhard et al. (1965) compared the interview responses of 1,356 white males convicted of sex offenses with those of two control groups. One control group consisted of white males who were not imprisoned. The second control group consisted of inmates convicted for crimes other than sexual offenses. Their data failed to demonstrate that sex offenders as a group were overly exposed to or overly responsive to sexual stimuli. The report of the President's Commission on Obscenity and Pornography (1970), which contains data from numerous research studies dealing with all aspects of the production, distribution, use and effects of sexually explicit material, also fails to show a significant relationship between pornography and criminal sexual behavior. Kercher and Walker (1973) studied 28 convicted rapists and 28 other inmates, who were shown one of a series of slides depicting sexual themes, while measures of penile volume, galvanic skin response (GSR) and subjective ratings were obtained. No significant differences were found between the groups on the penile volume measures, but the rapists displayed greater arousal on the GSR measure and gave more negative ratings to the sexual themes than did the nonrapists. Kercher and Walker conclude that the rapists did not show greater physiologic arousal to pornography than did the nonrapists. In addition, rapists tended to be rather conservative in their attitude toward sexuality.

REFERENCES

Bender, L., and Grugett, A. E.: A follow-up report on children who had atypical sexual experience, Am. J. Orthopsychiatry 22:825, 1952.

Blos, P.: Delinquency, in Lorand, S., and Schneer, H. I. (eds.): *Adolescents—Psychoanalytic Approach to Problems and Therapy* (New York: Harper-Hoeber, 1961).

Burton, L.: *Vulnerable Children: Three Studies of Children in Conflict: Accident Involved Children, Sexually Assaulted Children and Children with Asthma* (New York: Schocken Books, 1968).

Eissler, K. R.: Ego-psychological implications of the psychoanalytic treatment of delinquents, Psychoanal. Study Child 5:97, 1950.

Ferenczi, S.: Thalassa: a theory of genitality, Psychoanal. Q. 2:361, 1933.

Freud, S.: *The Etiology of Hysteria* (1896). Standard Edition, Vol. 3 (London: Hogarth Press, 1962), p. 187.

Freud, S.: *Hysterical Phantasies and Their Relationship to Bisexuality* (1908). Standard Edition, Vol. 9 (London: Hogarth Press, 1959), p. 155.

Gebhard, P. H., Gagnon, J. H., Pomeroy, W. B., and Christenson, C. V.: *Sex Offenders: An Analysis of Types* (New York: Harper and Row, 1965).

Hunter, G. R.: Rape: an organized approach to evaluation and treatment, Am. Fam. Physician 15:154, 1977.

Johnson, A. M.: Factors in the etiology of fixations and symptom choice, Psychoanal. Q. 22:475, 1953.

Kercher, G. A., and Walker, E. C.: Reactions of convicted rapists to sexually explicit stimuli, J. Abnorm. Psychol. 81:46, 1973.

Kinsey, A. C., Pomeroy, W. B., Martin, C. E., and Gebhard, P. H.: *Sexual Behavior in the Human Female* (Philadelphia: W. B. Saunders Co., 1953).

Klein, M.: *The Psychoanalysis of Children* (London: Hogarth Press, 1932).

Lafon, M. R., Trivas, J., and Pouget, R.: Aspects Psychologiques des attentats sexuels sur les enfants et les adolescents (Psychological aspects of sexual crime amongst children and adolescents), Ann. Med. Psychol. 2:865, 1958.

Landis, J. T.: Experiences of 500 children with adult sexual deviation, Psychiat. Q. [Suppl.] 30:91, 1956.

Moses, J.: Psychische Auswirkungen sexueller Angriffe bei Jungen Mädchen (Psychical consequences of sexual attacks upon young girls), Kinderheilkd. 40:542, 1932.

Perdue, W. C., and Lester, D.: Personality characteristics of rapists, Percept. Mot. Skills 35:514, 1972.

Rabinovitch, R. D.: Sexual psychopath, a symposium, J. Crim. Law Criminol. 43:592, 1953.

Rasmussen, A.: Die Bedeutung Sexueller Attentate auf Kinder unter 14 Jahren für die Entwicklung von Geisteskrankheiten und Charakteranomalien (The importance of sexual attacks on children less than 14 years of age for the development of mental diseases and character anomalies), Acta Psychiatr. Kbh. 9:351, 1934.

Report of the Commission on Obscenity and Pornography (New York: Bantam Books, 1970).

Seghorn, T. K.: Adequacy of ego functioning in rapists and pedophiles, Dissertation Abstracts International 31B:7613B, 1971.

Weiss, J., Rogers, E., Darwin, M., et al.: A study of girl sex victims, Psychiatr. Q. 29:1, 1955.

12/Child Abuse—Team Management

MALTREATMENT OF CHILDREN has existed throughout the ages. The realization of the importance of early development and proper upbringing has focused a great deal of attention on children in the last several decades. Children, however, live in the society of adults in a dependent role and are influenced by the frustrations, aggressions and sorrows experienced by the adults. The increasing rate of aggression and criminal activity on the part of adults is clearly reflected in the increasing rate of child abuse. It is estimated that at least 700 children are killed each year in the United States by parents and parent surrogates. This makes child abuse the leading cause of death among children, ahead of infectious diseases, leukemia and automobile accidents. The National Center for the Prevention and Treatment of Child Abuse in Denver estimated the incidence of child abuse cases at 60,000 in 1974 and 1,500,000 in 1975. Although some of this dramatic increase is due to better case-finding and reporting, the trend is certainly rising.

Maltreatment of children ranges from simple neglect to severe brutality. Many studies have tried to characterize parents who abuse their children. The findings reveal varying personality and emotional characteristics, such as immaturity, impulsiveness, self-centeredness, hypersensitivity and rapidity of reaction with poorly controlled aggression. Child abusers may be rigid, compulsive, passive-dependent and overcontrolled. Many of these characteristics are also found in nonabusive parents and are thus not specific to abusive parents. It is generally agreed that child abuse occurs in a highly emotionally charged state, at times during a temporary psychotic reaction. Although child abuse exists at all socioeconomic levels, children from low-income and welfare families are especially vulnerable. Many of these families are frequently besieged by problems of housing, nutrition, drugs, alcoholism, poor health, unstable marriages and sexual promiscuity. The parents are often isolated individuals, with few friends and little social life. Some of them are of borderline or low intelligence, which seems to make the care of a child, especially a problem child, very difficult. Many of the parents come from extremely deprived and neglected backgrounds themselves and are unable to trust or establish relationships with other people.

The Abused Child

Abused children are frequently problem children. They may be retarded, brain damaged, premature, hyperactive, colicky and temperamentally difficult to take care of. Perfectly healthy children may also be abused, as they may be unwanted by their parents. Certain personality characteristics in children may lead to abuse, since they may remind some parents of their hated sibling, a parent or some other person, or even some aspects of themselves that they dislike. Other contributory factors may be related to the events associated with the birth of the child, such as the death of a parent, financial disaster, the father's becoming an alcoholic or other calamities.

Circumstances of Abuse

It is generally agreed that abuse occurs in an atmosphere of intense parental anger and frustration. There are, however, occasional cases in which children have been abused in a premeditated manner in order to collect insurance money or to get rid of the child, who is felt to be too great a burden to care for. Child abuse also occurs in a state of severe parental depression or in some types of delusional psychosis. Child abuse is more likely to occur at certain stressful stages of child development, e.g., during the period of toilet training. There are some indications that certain parents themselves had difficulties in those stages of development but have repressed them. A child's problems bring out these repressed parental feelings, which interfere with the management of the child's difficulties.

Diagnosis of Child Abuse

Child abuse varies in degree of maltreatment from simple neglect to severe battering. A neglected child is rarely seen by a physician until he is suffering from some illness or infection or has some developmental problems. Such a child is more undernourished, with poorer skin hygiene, than would be the case if he were simply ill. His developmental milestones in physical, psychological and social areas are retarded. The Denver Developmental Test may be helpful as a screening test to determine the degree of retardation. The child may be quite irritable and unable to relate to adults in any meaningful manner. A severely neglected infant lies motionless in bed with little emotional expression, shows a fearful reaction when approached or touched, ignores the presence of adults and is frequently physically or mentally retarded.

The diagnosis of child battering depends heavily on a careful history, physical examination, x-ray findings and a high index of suspicion. Battering of a child ranges from simple bruises on various parts of the body to fractures of the bones and rupture of viscera. There is usually a great discrepancy between the history of how the child was injured and the extent of physical injury suffered by the child. The parents generally are afraid and tend to give all kinds of false stories. The parents, when interviewed separately, may give contradictory reports concerning the circumstances of the injury. Confrontation of the parents should be avoided initially, as it is likely to make them more defensive and less prone to cooperate with and participate in the plan of treatment and rehabilitation. Morris et al. (1964) have studied the attitudes of abusive parents toward their injured children. They found that such parents are evasive and contradictory concerning the circumstances of the injury and volunteer little information. They may appear angry and criticize the child for being injured. In general, there is an inappropriate verbal and emotional response. They seldom touch the injured child or look at him.

The parents are not likely to provide accurate information with regard to the history of multiple injuries treated at different hospitals. However, the presence of multiple scars and x-ray evidence of repeated trauma may be quite evident.

The physical examination of the child will reveal an unusual combination of injuries that cannot be explained by one set of circumstances, including bruises, fractures, hematomas, burns, rope marks and ruptured viscera. X-ray examination is important in all suspected cases of child abuse and should include the long bones, the ribs and the skull. X-rays may reveal several foci of reparative changes in various stages of healing. Other findings may include fragmentation of metaphyses, squaring of long bones, periosteal hemorrhages, calcification and presence of bone fragments and separation of epiphysis. Twisting of long bones may not be shown by any black or blue marks on physical examination but will have some of the above-mentioned findings on x-rays.

Kempe et al. (1962) reported that:

> Unless gross fractures, dislocations, or physical separation were produced, no signs of bone injury are found during the first week after a specific injury. Reparative changes may first become manifest about 12 to 14 days after the injury and can increase over the subsequent weeks, depending on the extent of initial injury and the degree of repetition. Reparative changes are more active in the growing

bones of children than in adults and are reflected radiologically in the excessive new bone reaction which may at times be confused with neoplastic changes.[1]

Other diagnostic categories, such as syphilis, scurvy, osteogenesis imperfecta, infantile cortical hyperostosis and congenital indifference to pain, need to be ruled out.

One cannot be certain of the nature of the injuries from the findings of the physical examination or x-rays. It is the total clinical picture derived from observation of the parents and the child, the history, physical examination and x-ray that should arouse suspicion of child abuse. A definite diagnosis of child abuse is a complex medical, social, psychological and legal determination and is arrived at by the combined efforts of the representatives of these disciplines.

Management

When negligence or abuse is suspected, the child should be admitted to a hospital for further investigation of physical injuries and/or for failure to thrive. Hospitalization provides protection for the child and the time necessary for a social and psychiatric evaluation of the family and the child. At the time of the child's admission, a social worker may be introduced to the family by the physician as a person who is interested in this type of problem. It is not necessary at this point to tell the parents that child abuse is suspected.

The social evaluation of the family for potential child abuse or neglect is a very difficult task. Abusing parents usually have a great deal of mistrust, hostility and anger toward the helping professions. Data gathered during interviews is generally not very conclusive, especially from denying and defensive parents. A home visit may be more helpful.

If the suspicion of child abuse is substantiated by the medical findings as well as by the social worker's evaluation, the case should be brought to the child abuse team of the hospital for a full discussion. The physician should tell the parents that the case is being brought to the hospital child abuse team for discussion because of the suspicion of child abuse or neglect. The physician should clarify his medical reasons for suspecting child abuse and his legal obligations to report such cases. He should also clarify the meaning of the report, together with the possible consequences. The purpose of reporting is to identify children who have been abused or neglected so that appropriate protective services can be provided to them. A child abuse team usually considers the following questions: Has abuse or negligence occurred? What is the potential for further abuse? Can the child return home without supportive services being made available to the

---

[1]Kempe et al.: J.A.M.A. 181:17, 1962.

family? If further services are required, can they be delivered on a voluntary basis or should there be immediate recourse to court?

The recommendations of the child abuse team should be discussed with the parents by the physician and the social worker. Some battering parents are likely to be hostile and verbally abusive when confronted. They may threaten legal reprisal or physical injury. A climate of violence or loss of control may prevail in such sessions. If, however, the physician and the social worker can demonstrate a concern for the parents as individuals and an interest in their problems as well as those of the child, the beginning of a working relationship can be established.

Psychiatric Evaluation of the Abused Child

Psychiatric evaluation of the victim should be carried out while the child is in the hospital. This evaluation should provide data concerning the factors that promote child abuse, including those inherent in the child. The evaluation should also determine the extent and the nature of the personality distortion, neurosis or psychosis that may have been induced by the abuse or neglect.

A retarded, brain-damaged, hyperkinetic or psychotic child may be quite difficult to cope with, especially for an unsophisticated parent. Such a child may provoke parental abuse and neglect. If such a diagnosis is indicated, a thorough evaluation should be made to provide the necessary services for the child and the supportive services for the parents. It is generally quite difficult to separate the primary problems of the child from the secondary problems caused by the abuse and neglect. An extensive developmental history is helpful in making such distinctions.

An abused child frequently develops a pattern of attention-seeking through negative actions, such as stubbornness, defiance or unacceptable behavior. Unfortunately, this pattern of attention-seeking creates a vicious circle in the family, where the child's negative behavior consistently precipitates parental abuse. Observing the child's behavior with the adults on the hospital ward (physicians, nurses, aides) may provide clues to the extent of this behavior pattern. An extremely negative child should be placed in a psychiatric inpatient setting for observation for a short period of time before being placed in a foster home or sent home. Immediate placement in a foster home without initial psychiatric intervention is frequently unsuccessful. These children have been known to be abused even by experienced foster parents, who then request the removal of the child, thus leading to multiple foster home placements for the child and the loss of good foster homes from the welfare department's roster.

Separation

If the child is to be placed out of his home, an initial work-up should be carried out with regard to the process of separation. No matter how rejecting the parents are or how unloving the child feels toward his parents, all members of the family mourn the separation and loss. Family sessions are very useful in assisting various members of the family to come to terms with their loss and with the subsequent alteration of their position in the family unit. It may be quite helpful for the child to know about and visit his foster parents in advance. Similarly, information regarding the child's eating habits, his daily routine, and his bedtime schedule allows foster parents to relate to the child more positively. The choice of other residential facilities for the child (such as temporary shelter homes, special schools, all-day care programs and psychiatric residential treatment centers) depends upon the extent and nature of the child's problems, the circumstances of the family and, most importantly, the availability of space in such facilities.

Court battles for custody of the child should be avoided if at all possible, since it appears to be an extremely traumatic situation for the parents and frequently destroys the possibility of establishing a positive, working relationship with the family. Courts require very detailed medical and social evidence to prove abuse and neglect beyond a reasonable doubt. Color photographs of the child taken at the time of admission are helpful in substantiating various pertinent medical findings. The social evaluation of the family should clearly indicate the psychological potential of the parents for further child abuse.

Follow-up Services

Each community should develop various follow-up services for abusive families. Whether the child is returned to his home or placed in the community, a regular follow-up visit is essential for the child and for the parents. Many hospitals and clinics code records of child abuse or use special colored folders so that these cases do not get lost in the shuffle. Most follow-up visits are to the departments of social service or psychiatry and rarely require medical examinations. However, children with developmental retardation or failure to thrive due to neglect require medical visits for the assessment of their development, nutrition and intercurrent illnesses. Important goals of follow-up services should include the provision of a safe physical and psychological environment for the child and rehabilitation of the parents so that the child can be returned to his family.

Several innovative approaches have been developed by various communities to help the parents through crises and to provide ongoing, continuous support. Such services include parents' anonymous groups, 24-hour emergency hot lines and 24-hour emergency nursery care for children. The services of social workers remain essential to the achievement of more lasting changes in these families.

Therapeutic work with the parents begins at the time the child is hospitalized. This is a very stressful time for the parents. Expressing kindness and support toward the parents will go a long way toward making them more amenable to later treatment. Therapeutic work with parents should be shared equally by physician, social worker and nurses. The social worker should make the parents feel accepted and should welcome them to the ward (even if the visits are supervised) and should inform them of the medical progress of their child. No direct or indirect attempt should be made to elicit a confession of guilt from the parents. Efforts should be concentrated instead on establishing a helpful working relationship with the family. This is a very difficult task, since most of these parents are suspicious, withdrawn and hostile toward the helping professional. Subsequent treatment should be directed toward strengthening the family unit by helping the parents deal with their unresolved conflicts and feelings of inadequacy and loneliness, thereby enhancing their capacity to provide good child care. Many of these families have multiple social and economic problems and require guidance in obtaining various services. There are frequent crises that require immediate intervention. The social worker should be available on these occasions to help the family through these difficult times. Sometimes, children have to be placed out of the home temporarily to give the parents time to cope with other problems. Each case is a challenge and requires a great many community resources.

Most states have created statewide central registries or data banks for child abuse and child neglect cases in order to keep track of families who are inclined to obtain medical and social services through different agencies at different times. The follow-up procedure should include the registration of these families.

Early Detection of High-Risk Cases

Full implementation of periodic screening, diagnosis and treatment could help identify high-risk children in poor families, who seem to have a larger proportion of abused and neglected children. Children of adolescent mothers, premature infants and illegitimate babies also fall into high-risk categories. It has been found that many parents had requested outside placement of their child before the abuse occurred, and all such requests should be investigated and given due attention. There is also a great deal of child abuse prevalent in the middle and upper classes. The responsibility for identifying abused children rests primarily with private pediatricians and internists. A more widespread understanding of the effects of neglect and abuse on children may facilitate early reporting of these cases.

Child Abuse Team

Most children's hospitals have multidisciplinary teams which review all suspected cases of child abuse and neglect. These teams are composed of a varying combination of hospital personnel, such as physicians, social workers, nurses, psychiatrists, administrators and chaplains. These teams should meet regularly or should be available on short notice. They should have a coordinator who, besides scheduling meetings, maintains the file of abuse cases, brings each case up for review on a periodic basis, collects information from other agencies involved and reports cases to local protective agencies. It is important to invite a representative of the local child protective agency to every meeting to keep the agency abreast of all new cases. Generally, it takes a while for these teams to function in a cohesive manner. Initial problems usually result from lack of understanding of mutual roles and ineffective communication. These teams should specify the role definition of each member and should operate with reciprocal trust and respect, remembering that making a diagnosis of child abuse and neglect is at present a community responsibility.

Legal Considerations

Every state in the union has statutory laws with regard to child abuse. Such laws are designed primarily to compel various professionals (physicians, nurses, social workers, lawyers) to report cases of child abuse and neglect to the proper local authorities. The statutes require notification when there is a reasonable suspicion that the injuries were inflicted rather than accidental. Most states have included immunity clauses to protect those who report child abuse cases from the civil and criminal liabilities which might otherwise ensue. Most child abuse laws also include a waiver of privileged communication, which allows the reporter to legally divulge confidential information to protective agencies. At least half of the states include a penalty clause or criminal sanction for failure to report child abuse–child neglect cases, and there have been a number of civil suits brought against physicians for failure to report these cases. Some suits have been settled out of court for sizable amounts.

It is estimated that only a small proportion of child abuse–child neglect cases are reported in spite of the mandatory reporting statutes. This chronic reporting failure may be attributed to several conscious and unconscious factors. Besides being negligent in making a proper diagnosis, physicians may be unwilling to get involved. This may be because of a busy schedule or from fear of deleterious economic impact on the practice. Lack of knowledge or misunderstanding of the law and its consequences also account for some proportion of unreported cases. The belief that reporting does not result in better services or appropriate legal action also deters many physicians from seeking appropriate protection for the abused child. Unfortunately, underreporting is one of the major factors responsible for the inadequacy of the present system of services that is available to victims and perpetrators of child abuse and child neglect.

Unconscious factors relate to the basic beliefs and the personality of the reporters. A physician, nurse or social worker may identify with the inflictor's impulsive emotions. This may impair his ability to recognize inflicted trauma and neglect in a child.

REFERENCES

Kempe, C. H., Silverman, F. N., Steele, B. F., et al.: The battered child syndrome, J.A.M.A. 181:17, 1962.

Morris, M. G., Gould, R. W., and Mathews, P. J.: Towards prevention of child abuse, Children 2:55, 1964.

13/Facing a Dying Child and His Family

ALMOST EVERY HOSPITAL has difficulty managing the terminally ill child. Although the medical and surgical treatments of disease make use of the newest drugs and the most sophisticated equipment, the emotional management of the dying child and his family is often handled in a primitive and awkward manner. Dealing with the emotional reactions of children and parents seems to be the hardest task for physicians. This task is frequently delegated to social workers or to other paraprofessionals, while the physician restricts himself to managing the medical problems.

The physician's avoidance may be understood in terms of his busy schedule, a lack of confidence in his ability to cope with the emotional situation, or sheer denial of death. The usual gratification of success is absent in treating a terminally ill child, and feelings of helplessness and ineffectuality commonly result in anger toward the patient, soon followed by guilt and emotional withdrawal and avoidance. In order to overcome feelings of helplessness, the physician may engage in unnecessary activity or needless treatment procedures.

Whatever the reason for the emotional detachment of the physician, however, it invariably results in poor management of the patient. Physicians cannot afford to delegate the management of terminally ill children to other personnel. They must understand the emotional reactions of terminally ill children and their parents and learn to deal with them.

Discussing the Diagnosis with Parents

Although making a correct diagnosis is always important, it is especially crucial in life-threatening situations. All the tests and consultations required to make a correct diagnosis should be obtained before discussing it with the parents.

In cases where a major part of the work-up is done by a specialist not known to the parents, the family physician should be present with the specialist to help present and interpret the diagnosis to the parents. The physician should realize the gravity of the news and its potential for arousing severe emotional reactions in the parents. If the diagnostic interview is handled properly, a great deal of difficulty can be avoided later on. A sufficient block of time (40 minutes to an hour) should be set aside for this interview, which should be conducted in a private room. Other members of the family may be invited to this interview if the parents so desire.

The interview should commence with a brief review of the history of the child's symptoms, followed by a discussion of the test results which led to the final diagnosis. The physician should attempt to reconstruct the logical series of deductions and inferences that he went through in arriving at his final diagnosis. He should then explain the steps of the diagnostic process to the parents in terminology they can understand. During the interview, the physician should pause at appropriate points to encourage and answer questions. The following additional points may be helpful in carrying out the diagnostic interview:

1. *Face the danger*. Giving bad news to parents is like confronting them with a danger. The interviewer can help the parents face this danger by encouraging them to verbalize their fear and apprehension and by accepting their emotional reactions as natural in this crisis situation.

2. *Discuss the tolerable*. The physician need not discuss both the diagnosis and the treatment plan in one interview. He should adjust the amount of information he gives the parents in accordance with their anxiety level. High anxiety slows down comprehension, and many parents block out a great deal of the information given to them during the first interview.

3. *Do not give false reassurances*. Although a supportive approach is necessary, giving parents blanket reassurances has serious pitfalls which sooner or later become apparent and which eventually undermine the parents' confidence in the physician.

4. *Do not encourage blame*. The physician should not encourage the parents to blame other professionals for inadequate or faulty diagnoses or for not doing an adequate work-up. Blaming previous doctors may make the current physician more acceptable to the parents, but it frequently interferes with the parents' acceptance of their feelings of anger and sadness.

5. *Discuss minor details*. When people are upset, tending to the myriad details of everyday life is harder, confusing and, at times, impossible. Parents may ask the physician's advice in dealing with situations which may seem minor but which are nevertheless important to them.

6. *Encourage the parents to accept help*. Feelings of guilt, fear and shame prevent some parents from accepting help from other people. To some, accepting help may be equivalent to loss of self-esteem.

Parental Reactions

Parents' responses to a life-threatening illness in their child vary with their cultural background, religious affiliation and financial status. Parental reaction may be minimal if the child has been quite sick before the diagnosis was made, since they may have been anticipating a serious illness and have in fact grieved in advance. The parents may also feel less shocked if the illness is relatively painless and the child accepts it bravely and fights against it courageously. If the symptoms of the illness had not been very serious earlier, however, the diagnosis may come as a shock to the parents. They may be stunned with disbelief. Some parents may continue talking about the child as if they had not heard the diagnosis. Some may show evidence of denial during the same session by mentioning future plans for the child. Others may begin to question the diagnosis and prognosis in a manner that indicates that they wish to talk the physician out of it. The physician, however, should not argue or feel intimidated. Sympathetic listening will facilitate the parents' acceptance of the diagnosis.

The parents' psychological reactions are designed to protect them from being overwhelmed with anxiety. The news of the fatal illness acts as an excessive sensory input, which cannot be handled adequately by most human beings and which causes the breakdown of coping mechanisms, resulting in physical responses such as shock, numbness, daze or fainting. In general, these are normal human reactions that occur in crisis situations. These physical responses block out further sensory input and give the organism a chance to regain its homeostasis. After the individual recovers from his initial physical reaction, cognitive and emotional mechanisms work together to protect him. Such psychological mechanisms as denial, distortion, rationalization and repression come into play. These mechanisms help the individual to process input slowly and at a rate that allows for assimilation. The nature and the intensity of these mechanisms depend upon the previous experience of the individual in similar situations.

During the first interview, most parents are not able to progress beyond the initial physical reaction. Their high level of anxiety makes it difficult for them to retain information. There is usually a long pause in the middle of the interview (usually after the diagnostic findings have been reviewed) during which the parents try to compose their thoughts. The physician should not terminate the interview at this time but should give the parents sufficient time to recover and ask further questions. A second interview should be scheduled in advance, to take place within a week, to discuss further questions about the disease and its management. A brief written summary of the disease and the test findings may be given to the parents to take home. The physician should not be offended if the parents ask for a second opinion. In fact, in certain circumstances, the physician himself may suggest that a second opinion be obtained and refer the parents to an appropriate specialized center. This suggestion, however, should be based upon the physician's assessment of the need for further investigation and not upon the desire to extricate himself from a difficult situation. Some parents may go from clinic to clinic in the hope of finding something less serious.

Common reactions of parents after the first interview include denial, distortion, rationalization, anger and guilt. Although these reactions are designed to protect the parents from being overwhelmed by grief and depression, their persistence delays the acceptance of the child's sickness and obstructs its adequate management.

The second interview with the parents is spent reviewing the possible causes of the disease and outlining a specific plan for its management. Etiologic considerations, such as genetic factors, pregnancy, birth, environment and child care, should be discussed both in general and with specific reference to the child. Questions about the outcome of future pregnancies may be handled by the physician or referred for genetic counseling. The discussion of the treatment should include instructions for general management (social, psychological, educational and physical), medication (including expected major side effects) and the management of relapses should they occur.

The initial acknowledgment of the disease frequently arouses anger in parents. This anger may be directed at members of the treatment team, other family members or the sick child. One or both parents may begin to get angry at the other over minor matters and may scold their children for minor misbehavior. They may call the doctor in the middle of the night to complain about a new pain their child is having. Members of the treatment team should not take the hostility and anger expressed toward them personally. They should, however, confront such parents with their anger in a sympathetic way: "We realize that you are going through a very difficult time, we are doing all we can, but your anger is not likely to accomplish anything constructive and may alienate some members of the team." Anger at the child may be expressed indirectly by undue restrictions and overprotection. The parents may confine the child to bed, while the physician's instructions were only to avoid overexertion on the part of the child. Similarly, other restrictions may be carried to extremes. Other children in the family may also be subjected to restrictions and overprotection "for their own safety."

The anger reaction usually lasts a few days and is then replaced by guilt and self-blame, although some parents may continue projecting the blame on to other people. Sources of guilt frequently arise from actual or fantasied causes of the disease which may be related to genetics, pregnancy, birth and various aspects of child care. The presence of an actual genetic etiology in the child's disease causes the most guilt. Grief and depression may set in soon after the diagnostic work-up, especially if the child's condition deteriorates quickly.

Discussing the Diagnosis with the Child

Should a young child be informed of the diagnosis and the prognosis for his disease?

Who should tell the child? And what should be said?

Realizing how shocking the diagnosis can be, many parents try to spare their sick child the further suffering that knowledge of the diagnosis would bring. "Ignorance is bliss," they rationalize. "The child may not understand it anyway," or "He is likely to distort the information in all sorts of ways and worry over it all the time." They worry about the child's emotional reactions to the diagnosis and his inability to cope with them. Some clinicians have similar views and do not like to discuss the diagnosis with the child. Other clinicians (Friedman, 1967, 1964; Green, 1967) believe that the child should be told and emphasize the relief experienced by children who are informed of their diagnosis. They point out that mothers who keep the diagnosis a secret use all their available energy to maintain this state of secrecy and cannot devote themselves to the more positive and important task of supporting the child. Such secretiveness also interferes with the child's developing a sincere, trusting relationship with his parents, a relationship the child must have if he is to deal with his fears and anxiety.

Bluebond-Langer (1978) argues against secrecy. She points out that a terminally ill child knows that he is dying well before death becomes imminent. She describes in great detail how the dying child learns about his illness through information acquired from multiple sources. He gradually and progressively arrives at the conclusion that he is dying by putting together information about the disease, hospital functions and special treatments, reactions of various members of the family toward him, reactions of doctors, nurses and other caretakers and information from other sick children. She asserts that leukemic children acquire this information in five stages.

During the first stage, children learn that they are suffering from a serious illness. Some of them also learn the name of the disease that they are suffering from and the names of the drugs that they are being treated with. During the second stage, most children acquire knowledge about the side effects and other consequences of their medication. During the third stage, the child learns the special procedures used in administering the drugs and in treating their side effects. The fourth stage is marked by the child's realization that his disease is marked by "a series of relapses and remissions," which occur despite the drugs and other treatment procedures. During the fifth stage, the child realizes that there is no magic drug that will cure his disease and that the cycle of relapses and remissions will end in death.

Corresponding to the above five stages of acquisition of knowledge about their disease, children defined themselves as:

1. Seriously ill
2. Seriously ill and will get better
3. Always ill and will get better
4. Always ill and will never get better
5. Dying

If Bluebond-Langer's observations are correct, it would be foolhardy for parents or physicians to hide the diagnosis and prognosis from the child, letting him suffer alone with his fears and anxieties at the very time when he needs and seeks strength and support.

What in fact should the child be told about his diagnosis and prognosis?

Once it is agreed that the diagnosis of the disease should be shared with the child, further questions arise: What does a young child understand about death and dying? How can we explain this difficult concept so that there is no distortion and no fantasy elaboration?

Little is known about the exact manner in which children acquire the concept of death. However, several developmental theories provide guidelines that are helpful in understanding this issue.

Children's Concepts of Death

Death is defined as a final separation—a dead person leaves forever and will not be seen again in this world. The development of intelligence and emotions helps children acquire partial concepts of death at different ages. It seems that full comprehension of death as defined is not acquired until 10–12 years of age. This statement may seem contrary to observations made of much younger children, some of whom seem to comprehend death fairly well. However, studies of cognitive and emotional development indicate that death is not fully comprehended until preadolescent or early adolescent years (Nagy, 1959; Anthony, 1972).

During the first 3 years of life, the child is very dependent upon his parents. There is a progressive separation and individuation from the parents. The usual emergence of separation anxiety in 10-month-old children may be experienced by the child in the same way that the death of a loved one is experienced by adults.

Children between 3 and 5 experience separation from parents by going to school or preschool. This experience may be extremely anxiety-provoking for children who have not been well prepared for it, and some of them develop school phobia. During these years, children also show curiosity about dead flowers, leaves and animals, which contributes to the cognitive understanding of death.

In school-age children between 5 and 10, death is personified. Children hold their breath while passing a cemetery in order not to be spooked (taken possession of by dead spirits). Religious teachings help them to conceptualize the meaning of death and what happens to people after death. Death anxiety, commonly experienced by children around 8–10 years of age, is heightened in cases where a death has occurred in the family or the child has experienced the death of a beloved pet. During the early school years, dying is frequently equated with going away. Although an 8-year-old child may cognitively understand the difference between dying and going away, an emotional comprehension of this difference does not seem to be acquired until 10–12 years of age. Children also associate death with extreme pain, torture or severe trauma. A full comprehension of death by a child may arouse the same emotional reactions as separation anxiety.

The evolution of death concepts parallels the development of cognitive abilities. Piaget (1962) divides the development of cognitive functions into four major stages: (1) sensory-motor stage, (2) preoperational stage, (3) concrete operational stage and (4) formal operational stage.

The sensory-motor stage of intellectual development occurs during the first 2 years of a child's life. During the first 3 months, the infant repeats simple acts (e.g., repetitive opening and closing of fists) for his own sake, without much intent and purpose. By 4 months of age, he uses his motor movements to produce interesting results in the environment, such as knocking over a pillow in order to obtain a toy hidden underneath it. By 1 year of age, the child begins active trial-and-error experimentation, e.g., a child who has learned to knock over a pillow with his fist to get a toy may then attempt to knock it over with his foot or may use a rattle for the same purpose. By 18–24 months of age, the child appears to have developed some primitive form of imagery or memory, which he utilizes in problem-solving.

During the preoperational stage (2–6 years), symbolic functions begin to appear. At the sensory-motor level, the games were nothing but physical exercise. Now they become symbolic play, representing something by means of something else. Also, the child learns to imitate. The imitation occurs not only in the presence but also in the absence of the original object. Development of language facilitates symbolic expression.

During the concrete operational stage (7–11 years), the child begins to organize the world around him by classifying objects according to their similarities and differences and by arranging objects according to their sizes and weights. He is capable of planning and carrying out a series of actions.

During the formal operational stage, which begins around 12 years of age, the child begins to reason not only on the basis of objects but also on the basis of hypotheses and propositions. Adolescents begin to think of various ways of solving a problem and then check each method and solution for its probable validity. The adolescent's thoughts become self-consciously deductive. He can think in terms of hypotheses and propositions that may be fanciful and independent of the given reality.

One cannot talk about death to a child without first understanding his ideas and concepts of death and illness. Thus, the first thing a physician must do is to ask the child what he thinks about his illness, how sick he thinks he is. Inquire about his perception of the causes of his illness and his fears. In most cases, all the physician has to do is to correct some misapprehensions to relieve a great deal of the child's anxiety and fears. Although it is not necessary to mention death with young children, some of them may ask the physician if they are going to die. Before answering this question, one must first know how that particular child conceives of death. One may ask a young child, "Do you know what death is?" or "Why are you afraid of death?" Some children fear they will suffer severe pain or will be mutilated before they die. The physician should try to assure the child that he is doing his best to make the child better, but that if the child is going to die, he will not be mutilated. Some physicians or parents may even want to ask the child his last wishes before he dies.

Older children, although aware of their terminal illness, are frequently afraid to discuss it. The physican or parents should promote discussion of the diagnosis and prognosis of their illness.

Emotional Reactions of Children

A great many of the emotions expressed by dying children are associated with the pain, discomfort and restrictions caused by their illness. Imminent or possible new procedures and operations keep some children in a perpetual state of fear of pain and mutilation. Preschool children may express anger toward their parents and other adults, including doctors and nurses, for not relieving their discomfort and pain. Some school-age children associate sickness with punishment. They feel that some of their acts, desires and thoughts are unacceptable and bad and see their sickness as the consequence.

The emotions of children frequently parallel the emotions expressed by their parents. Parental feelings of sadness and depression are easily communicated to the child in overt and covert ways. Children who have learned that they are dying feel afraid, lonely and sad if not supported by their parents.

Young adolescents are perhaps the most sensitive to death fears. They fully comprehend the irreversibility of death, and many are quickly able to deduce the severity of their condition. Not only does their illness represent the curtailment of their freedom and the possibility of ultimate extinction, but for some it also represents a dreadful adult retaliation against their strivings for independence. Their illness may thus engender intense anger and guilt and may produce a total denial of all that is happening.

The adolescent who is dying is liable to be rejected by his peer group. The other teenagers in his crowd withdraw emotionally when they are faced with the impending death of one of their own age group. These young men and women are working very hard to establish their own self-sufficiency and independence. They are building their strengths and solidifying their own opinions. Death, especially the death of a friend or someone their own age, makes them intensely aware of their vulnerability and fragility. Most adolescents cannot tolerate this kind of open awareness of their very human fragility. They tend to pull back from anyone who symbolizes fragility. They are uncomfortable with the maimed and the disfigured and are unbearably uncomfortable when they deal with someone their own age who is dying.

The adolescent who is facing death thus tends to be very lonely. He feels neglected by his parents and isolated from his peers. He struggles against the dependent role forced upon him by his illness. He may ridicule other patients who are handicapped to bolster his self-esteem and deny his own feelings of mutilation. The young adolescent must convince himself of his self-sufficiency and independence. If he turns to his parents for support, understanding and comfort, he may feel that he is surrendering his independence and that he is submitting to their punishment. The lonely, dying adolescent may violently reject his parents, his family and the adult members of the treatment team—not because he is without desperate need of their understanding and support but because he longs so intensely for their warmth and caring that he cannot allow himself to admit to these feelings, so reminiscent of the dependent infant. He wishes so desperately to be cared for and protected that he dreads losing control over himself. He longs for understanding but so greatly fears the loss of his new independence that he has to force people away. Gifts may be tossed away unopened. Letters may be left unread to show how self-sufficient he really is.

As the adolescent becomes weaker and unable to care for himself, he may then accept, without too much sign of resistance, the attention of his parents and family.

How Should a Terminally Ill Child be Treated?

There is often a tendency on the part of adults, including parents and relatives, to restrict and overprotect a child suffering from a life-threatening illness. This overly protective attitude on the part of adults may help them to work through their own anger and guilt, but it is likely to make the sick child quite unhappy. A bedridden, demanding and irritable child is not a happy child. Happiness in children comes from a positive and trusting relationship with parents and from feelings of accomplishment. The child should be allowed to be as physically active as possible. He should continue his education by attending a regular or special school. If he misses too many school days, his school work may be brought to him while he is in the hospital or at home. Social and recreational activities should be promoted with family members as well as with peers. A child in the hospital should be encouraged to write to his friends, to keep in touch and to maintain contact with them.

The family should maintain its traditional style of discipline. A sick child who is used to a certain type of discipline may feel guilty if he is allowed to get away with too many things. Insofar as possible, he should take part in household chores and not be allowed to act abusively or aggressively to others.

Reactions of Siblings

Parents frequently try to overprotect the healthy siblings of a dying child by keeping them ignorant of the diagnosis and the prognosis of the disease. However, excessive parental preoccupation with the dying child makes the healthy siblings feel neglected. They may become angry, demanding and aggressive. Older siblings who become aware of the life-threatening nature of the illness may nevertheless feel upset and resentful over the secretive attitude of their parents. They may also feel angry at the dying sibling for destroying the family's fun. "Nobody laughs anymore. Everybody is always quiet and serious. They all seem to be afraid of something," remarked one 10-year-old sibling. These feelings may in turn arouse guilt, which may lead to self-blame, sadness or acting-out behavior.

Some children, observing their sick brother or sister mutilated from operations or suffering from side effects of drug treatment, become afraid of catching the illness.

The physican should encourage the parents to hold family discussions at frequent intervals. The parents should share their understanding of the child's illness with the siblings and allow all members of the family to express their fears and feelings. This is a crisis situation not only for the parents but for the whole family. Children are much more cooperative and have fewer problems if they share the crisis with their parents. The exclusion of healthy siblings from information about and discussion of the dying child only causes them to suffer in silence. Furthermore, parents lose the opportunity that a crisis situation provides to develop a closer and more honest relationship within the family.

Home Care for a Dying Child

It is ironic that the sick child is separated from his parents and his family at the very time when he most needs their support. Certainly, the nature of the disease and the specialized care provided in hospitals warrants the child's removal to the hospital, but little attention has been given to developing community resources outside the hospital that could help the dying child to be cared for at home. There are indications that many very sick children do much better at home. They are happier and require less medication for pain. There are some parents who, for various reasons, may feel inadequate and apprehensive about taking a very sick child home. There are others, however, who wish to have their child at home during the last few weeks or days of his life.

Under what circumstances should a physician allow a sick child to be treated at home? Although it is difficult to evaluate the motivation of parents who make such requests, most parents wish to do something special for the child and to be with him in his last days. The decision should be based on two major factors: (1) suitability of the home for the care of the sick child and (2) availability of competent 24-hour nursing care. The suitability of the home may be judged by the physical space available for the sick child, preferably a separate room to avoid the resentment of other siblings, and the presence of one of the parents or other adult at all times. The physician should investigate, at least to some degree, the feelings of other members of the family toward the home care of the sick child. The availability of competent nursing care on a round-the-clock basis is extremely important.

In their home care project, Martinson and associates (1976) found that the first days, and particularly the first day at home with the sick child, were "almost overwhelming" for the parents. This is the time during which the parents feel most helpless and need the greatest support from the nurse and the physician. The preparation for home care needs to be started in the hospital, where parents are taught various procedures which they will do themselves at home. Visiting nurses should also let the parents carry out the procedures by themselves under their supervision. This is what gives the parents most confidence and reduces their anxiety in taking care of their sick child. The parents should also be informed of the complications that may occur, such as hemorrhage, infection and coma, and should be taught how to manage them. Most parents prefer knowing about the worst complications in advance rather than facing them unprepared.

One of the most persistent problems identified in home care is the control and effects of pain on the child and his family (Graner, 1976). The most frequent responses of parents to their child's pain were feelings of helplessness, anger, guilt and powerlessness to sufficiently relieve, control or prevent pain.

Psychologically, a great benefit is derived from home care of a dying child. Every member of the family has a chance to do some good for the dying child and thus feels satisfied. There are less prolonged periods of grief, and frequently less guilt is felt. For the dying child, it is much less painful and usually a more secure environment in which to die.

Interviews with Parents after the Child's Death

The parents should be informed immediately of the child's death, irrespective of the time of day or night. This information should be given by the doctor who has provided the primary care to the child and who is aware of the circumstances of death. If the parents are already in the hospital and waiting, they may hear about the child's death first from a nurse or ward secretary, but they should be told that the physician will see them soon. This interview should be given high priority by the physician, and the parents should not be kept waiting for any length of time.

If the child dies after the parents have gone home, a nurse or ward secretary may call to tell them that the physician wants to see them. Most parents realize these calls have been prompted by the worsening of the child's condition or his death. When the child is suffering from a life-threatening illness, death is expected, and the parents may ask the caller if the child has died. The answer should be given directly and honestly, "Yes, Mrs. Jones, we feel very sad about it." It is even better if the physician in charge can anticipate the gravity of the child's condition and ask somebody to call the parents in advance while he is trying to revive the child or carry out some other emergency procedure. Parents should be prepared in advance to receive such telephone calls.

The purpose of the interview with the parents after the child's death is twofold: first, to describe and answer the parents' questions about the circumstances of death and, second, to obtain permission for necropsy (which most hospitals require). This interview should be carried out in a separate room where the parents do not feel inhibited about grieving and crying. The physician should allow ample time for the parents to express their grief. It is not necessary to say anything while the parents are weeping. Waiting silently and patiently usually helps the parents to hold their tears long enough to ask some questions. This is not the occasion for the physician to apologize or express his shortcomings or his inability to save the child. There is nothing the physician can say in this regard that would minimize the parents' grief. Most parents desire information about the circumstances and causes of death. The physician should present this information in the simplest possible way and should allow sufficient time to answer questions.

When the death occurs in the newborn nursery, the obstetrician or pediatrician should contact the father first and, after dealing with his feelings, should decide who is to tell the mother. Some fathers may prefer talking to their wives themselves. The parents may or may not ask to see the baby. The physician should honor the parents' wishes in this matter and should not prevent them from seeing the baby if they so wish.

The request for necropsy should be made after the physician feels that the parents have no further questions about the circumstances of the death. Some parents may bring up this issue themselves and provide the physician with the opportunity to discuss it further. The reasons for necropsy should be explained: that it often contributes to medical knowledge, permits an evaluation of current medical practice and may provide answers to some puzzling aspects of the child's illness. Many parents fear that necropsy will mutilate the child's body. Some parents may wish to consult other family members before making a decision. The physician himself may suggest this if he observes hesitation and resistance on the part of the parents. If the parents refuse permission, the physician should accept their decision and not attempt to compel them to change their minds. The information obtained from necropsy does not offset the negative effects of the feelings of guilt and helplessness that follow when permission for a necropsy is obtained through intimidation.

Before terminating the interview, the physician should ask the parents if they need any help with funeral arrangements. If they do, the parents can be referred to the social service department of the hospital.

The physician should schedule a second interview a few weeks after the death of the child. This interview should focus on the bereavement process of the family. The parents are normally depressed at the time of the second interview. Their patterns of sleeping and eating are disturbed. Their daily routine and work also suffer to a moderate degree. The physician, however, should try to determine if the parents are experiencing excessive denial or guilt and whether they have shared the information about the child's death with the siblings. It is not uncommon for parents to hide the child's death, especially from younger siblings, by fabricating stories of the deceased child's going away to some other place or staying in the hospital for a long period of time. Although the death of a sibling has different meanings at different ages, hiding death from a young child may make him fearful that he himself may be sent away to a hospital or some other place.

The parents' guilt may be related to their own perceived contribution to a child's death. The physician should encourage them to discuss their thoughts about the causes of the child's death. This will allow the physician to correct parental misconceptions.

The time required to complete the mourning process varies from person to person. However, mourning is frequently regarded as abnormal if it is continued with moderate severity one year after the death. Individuals still in mourning after one year may have deep-seated feelings of anger and guilt that are not resolved by the passage of time. They may require psychiatric consultation and perhaps psychotherapy to work through these feelings.

Health Care Personnel

The task of the physician and other health care personnel is to continue battling the forces that cause the deterioration of the body and its death. Many children with terminal illnesses are kept alive, sometimes at a vegetative functional level, in the hope that a new cure will soon be found. Paradoxically, this often leads to aloofness and emotional detachment on the part of health care personnel.

An emergency, such as a serious accident, demands that the physician utilize all his skills to revive and save the individual. Most emergency procedures require a high level of technical skill and some degree of emotional detachment. Unfortunately, young physicians are frequently reproached for their emotional detachment.

For the purpose of management, the human body has to be compartmentalized and understood in terms of various mechanical and chemical functions. Human emotions, however, cannot be understood in the same manner, since the physiology and chemistry of human emotions are still at a primitive level of understanding. Most people respond to other people's emotions by empathizing with them. Since management of an emergency situation requires some degree of emotional detachment, this manner of responding to other people's emotions is generally not available to the physician in such a situation.

Personnel caring for terminally ill children face a similar type of problem. Although they are not dealing with an emergency situation, they have to reach into their own feelings about death in order to respond to the dying child's emotions. This is the most difficult task that health personnel face in the care of a terminally ill child. The denial of their own feelings about death is manifested by such clichés as, "Don't get involved," "Involvement with dying children interferes with their management," "Overinvolvement hurts you later on." Such advice is frequently given by colleagues and spouses who must bear the brunt of their grief and hurt.

Perhaps physicians should consider the dying syndrome as a condition secondary to all terminal illnesses. It can then be defined as consisting of definite emotional and physiologic manifestations. Once it is recognized, we will learn how to respond to these manifestations, perhaps without having to bring our own empathy into play. However, there is no guarantee that learning about the dying syndrome would free us from facing our own feelings about death. After all, this is one of the most common syndromes and the one we will experience ourselves someday.

REFERENCES

Anthony, S.: *The Discovery of Death in Childhood and After* (New York: Basic Books Inc., 1972).

Bluebond-Langer, M.: *The Private Worlds of Dying Children* (Princeton, N.J.: Princeton University Press, 1978).

Friedman, S. B.: Care of the family of the child with cancer, Pediatrics 40:498, 1967.

Friedman, S. B.: The child with leukemia and his parents, Cancer 4:73, 1964.

Graner, A.: The effects of pain on child, parent and health professional, in Martinson, I. M. (ed.): *Home Care for the Dying Child* (New York: Appleton-Century-Crofts, 1976).

Green, M.: Care of the dying child, Pediatrics 40:492, 1967.

Martinson, I. M. (ed.): *Home Care for the Dying Child* (New York: Appleton-Century-Crofts, 1976).

Nagy, M. H.: The child's view of death, in Feifel, H. (ed.): *The Meaning of Death* (New York: McGraw-Hill, 1959).

Piaget, J.: The stages of the intellectual development of the child, Bull. Menninger Clin. 26:120, 1962.

14/Management of Irate Parents

First Situation

"Dr. Shore, please come to the emergency department," announced the hospital paging system.

Dr. Shore, who is the head of the emergency department and a very busy man, is known to be quite adept in dealing with irate parents. As he arrived in the emergency department, one of the nurses told him that Mr. Mosely was very angry and upset about the medical care of his daughter. Dr. Shore spent a few minutes looking through the medical chart, then walked to the waiting area where Mr. Mosely was standing near the receptionist.

Dr. Shore: "Mr. Mosely, I am Dr. Shore, head of the emergency department. May I talk to you about this problem in my office?"

Mr. Mosely: "I am very upset, these people here. . . ." "Please come to my office," interrupted Dr. Shore. "I would prefer to discuss this in the office."

Dr. Shore turned around and walked toward his office. Mr. Mosely hesitated briefly but then followed the doctor. Many people may resist accompanying the doctor to his office because they may feel that their angry outburst is more effective in the waiting room, and they feel safer and more comfortable in the presence of other people. Some people may also be afraid of their own impulses, fearing they may lose control if they are alone with the doctor. However, the doctor should not allow the angry parent to elect any other option and should insist that the parent follow him to his office if he wants to continue the discussion.

It is rare that a parent will continue making a scene in the waiting area after this offer. Occasionally, if the parent does not follow the doctor, he is likely to calm down by himself. In such situations, the doctor may come back and tell the parent that he will be available should the parent wish to talk with him and will inform the receptionist accordingly.

Once in the office, "Please have a seat," invited Dr. Shore politely, pointing to a specific chair.

Mr. Mosely hesitated again but sat down, still looking very angry and sitting on the edge of the chair. Anger and tension were apparent on his face and in his body posture.

It is important to note the physical manifestations of anger and tension at the beginning of the interview. The changes in these manifestations are good indicators of how the interview is progressing and whether the anger and tension are dissipating.

Dr. Shore: "Could you please tell me the problem that you are having with this hospital?"

Mr. Mosely: "It is very difficult to describe. People here don't seem to understand you. Nurses are extremely impolite. Doctors are inconsiderate. It is just the whole place that's bad."

Brief silence

"Let me give you a specific example. I brought my daughter here two days ago. She was very sick with a 103 degree fever and was coughing a lot. We had to wait for 2 hours before she was seen. The doctor examined her in a cursory way and prescribed aspirin. It did not help. In fact, she got worse—more coughing, vomiting and not eating. But the doctors feel that these are minor symptoms, that she is basically okay and that I should not have brought her back here."

Silence

OBSERVATION: Dr. Shore noticed that Mr. Mosely was sitting back in the chair. His face looked less angry, and his body posture was less tense. He decided to promote further ventilation by Mr. Mosely.

Dr. Shore: "Please go on."

Mr. Mosely: "There is really not much more to say. I am a very busy man. I work 2 jobs. My wife also works in the evening. We can't afford our children being sick for long periods. The staff here think we're being neglectful parents. The truth of the matter is that they haven't treated our daughter properly and have been negligent in their work."

Silence

OBSERVATION: It appeared that Mr. Mosely did not want to go on and expected some response from Dr. Shore. The doctor also noticed that although Mr. Mosely's last sentence was uttered in a somewhat louder voice, he appeared relaxed and that the anger had drained from his face.

Dr. Shore: "We try to teach all our staff to be thoughtful and considerate, but we are not always successful."

Mr. Mosely: "I don't expect anything fancy. All I care about is that my child is treated properly."

OBSERVATION: Dr. Shore's comment was general and was related to the nature of the situation. He did not, however, blame particular personnel or admit to their having made mistakes. In fact, it is impossible to know in such situations whether and why somebody mistreated Mr. Mosely.

Dr. Shore: "I appreciate your concern about your daughter. How do you suggest we handle this situation now?"

Mr. Mosely: "I really don't want any privileged treatment."

Silence

OBSERVATION: Solicitation of suggestions for handling the problem is an important part of the interview. Such suggestions should be requested only after the anger and tension have dissipated, and the situation has been sufficiently clarified.

Mr. Mosely: "I just want somebody to examine her carefully."

Dr. Shore: "Fine. Would you mind going back to the waiting area? I will convey your concern to the examining doctor."

Some physicians might feel quite angry at such a father, who appears self-centered and seems to care only about himself, especially in an emergency room situation where nurses and doctors are frequently busy. They feel like telling the parent off or even ejecting him from the emergency room for being disruptive and overly demanding. But one has to remember that people are different in their perceptions of inconvenience and lack of courtesy. Some feel more slighted by minor situations than others do. Some are more aggressive, assertive and complaining than others. These are normal variations among normal people. Learning to deal with their anger and complaints is an integral part of the delivery of medical care.

Mr. Mosely's complaint is a simple but frequently occurring one in many centers of health care delivery. More complex situations arise when unnecessary procedures are carried out, especially when they cause some harm to the child. Many parents find it difficult to compromise in such situations, and their anger may lead to malpractice suits.

Second Situation

A man came to a psychiatric outpatient clinic and expressed his anger to the receptionist, threatening to sue the hospital and demanding to see the head of the psychiatry service immediately. The director happened to be available and responded to the receptionist's call.

Dr. Byrd: "Hello Mr. Max, I'm Dr. Byrd, director of the psychiatry service. What can I do for you?"

"What kind of hospital are you guys running here? Nobody seems to know what they're doing," Mr. Max boomed in an angry tone.

Dr. Byrd: "Please come to my office; we can talk about this there."

Mr. Max followed Dr. Byrd without further comment. Once in the office, he exploded: "It took me a long time to get used to the idea that my daughter needed hospitalization for several weeks for a psychiatric work-up. Now they tell me that there is no room for her and that she can best be worked up on an outpatient basis."

Silence

OBSERVATION: Mr. Max's face was still flushed and his muscles were tense. He was still standing despite the offer from the doctor to sit down. Dr. Byrd took a chair for himself and moved another chair toward Mr. Max, gesturing for him to sit down.

Mr. Max sat down reluctantly, then continued: "My wife and I have been pushed around by different doctors during the past 5 years. Nobody seems to know what our daughter's problem is. Some tell us she is retarded. Others think she has some kind of neurologic disease. Now, psychiatrists say she has an emotional problem. I don't know who to believe."

Silence

Dr. Byrd: "I can see that all this must be very confusing to you."

Mr. Max: "It isn't only the doctors. Her teacher and speech therapist also tell us different stories. They think she is bright but has no motivation and doesn't apply herself. They are inclined to blame us for babying her too much. I don't think they have the slightest idea of the time and effort we spend on her at home."

Silence

Dr. Byrd: "Please go on."

Mr. Max cleared his throat and began to talk in a much softer voice. "She is a very difficult child to care for. My wife and I spend a great deal of time with her, playing with her, teaching her. After she was born, her pediatrician told us that she had a small head and was going to be retarded. She was a pretty baby. We didn't believe the pediatrician. We have spent a great deal of time with her. She appears quite smart in some areas but has difficulty in other areas. We don't know what the problem really is."

OBSERVATION: The anger in Mr. Max's face had gone. He appeared relaxed, rather sad-looking and depressed.

Dr. Byrd: "I agree with you that this confusion about the nature of your daughter's problem should be clarified as soon as possible."

OBSERVATION: Dr. Byrd was aware that a previous neurologic work-up had resulted in a diagnosis of microcephaly. The parents had been reluctant to accept the diagnosis of mental retardation. Their reluctance had been reinforced by the well-meaning but unwise comments of some professionals. This is not an uncommon situation with parents of retarded youngsters.

Mr. Max continued in the same soft voice: "I guess we know what the problem is, but there is this nagging feeling inside us that forces us to believe that she is not retarded and may be trained to live a happy, normal life."

Dr. Byrd: "We will be happy to do everything we can to explore this possibility."

Mr. Max: "I would like to know why Dr. James (head of the inpatient service) changed his mind about hospitalization."

Dr. Byrd: "Did he say anything to you about this?"

Mr. Max: "Yes, he talked to my wife and said that the diagnosis was fairly clear and nothing was to be gained from hospitalization."

Dr. Byrd: "But you still have some questions about the diagnosis?"

Mr. Max: "We really don't care about the diagnosis. We know she has weaknesses but she also has unrealized strengths and potential. All we are interested in is learning how to help her achieve these strengths and potentials."

Dr. Byrd: "And you believe that this goal can be achieved by hospitalization?"

Mr. Max: "Yes, I believe that you people could observe her for a few weeks and find out what she is really like. Then you could give us suggestions on how to handle her."

Dr. Byrd: "That seems reasonable. Have you told this to Dr. James?"

Mr. Max: "Not really. We were more concerned about the correct diagnosis when we talked with him."

Dr. Byrd: "Would you like me to arrange another meeting with Dr. James so that you can discuss with him what you hope to accomplish from this hospitalization?"

The father agreed. A meeting was held with both parents and Dr. James. The child was hospitalized for observation and behavior modification.

Causes of Anger in Parents

Guilt

Feelings of guilt are the most frequent response of parents to the illness of their child. In one case, a 10-year-old boy who was seriously injured while running away from home after an argument with his father, the father felt extremely guilty and spent a great deal of time taking care of his son. He expressed anger whenever he felt his son was not receiving the best medical care.

There are many other situations that may arouse guilt feelings in parents. The presence of genetic disorders in their children makes many parents feel guilty of transmitting a defective gene to their child. Similarly, the appearance of a serious illness in a child may arouse all kinds of guilt feelings in the parents. The parents may focus upon some period in the child's life during which they neglected their child, or they may blame themselves for not providing better medical care before the disease was detected. Some parents may regard the child's illness as punishment for their own sins.

Personality Disorders

Personality disorders are characterized by deeply ingrained maladaptive patterns of behavior often existing since early adolescence. Adults with personality disorders are encountered in every clinic, and dealing with them is usually an exasperating experience. Physicians can minimize their exasperation with such adults by learning to recognize these disorders.

ANTISOCIAL PERSONALITY.—These adults are incapable of significant loyalty to others. They tend to be grossly selfish, callous, irresponsible, impulsive and unable to feel guilt or learn from either experience or punishment. Their frustration tolerance is low, and their past history often reveals alcoholism, drug addiction and unlawful activities.

HYSTERICAL PERSONALITY.—This disorder is more common among women. Hysterical women are easily excitable, emotionally unstable, self-dramatizing and overreactive. They are attention-seeking and often seductive. They may also be vain, self-centered and dependent on others and often have a long history of illnesses that defy diagnosis.

PASSIVE-AGGRESSIVE PERSONALITY.—These adults are very difficult to deal with because they are often obstructive, procrastinating and intentionally inefficient or stubborn. Their behavior is an expression of an underlying hostility that they dare not express openly because it is directed toward something or someone on whom they are overly dependent.

INADEQUATE PERSONALITY.—These adults respond ineffectually to emotional, social, intellectual and physical demands. Their adaptation is inadequate, and they are inept, socially unstable and use poor judgment.

Some adults with personality disorders are very adept at causing conflict among the hospital or clinic staff by pitting members against one another. Sympathetic staff members are likely to hear a description of the injustices perpetrated by the rest of the staff. Frequently, these adults may succeed in enlisting self-appointed advocates who agree to take up their client's cause against the alleged maltreatment.

Genuine Reasons

Sometimes, given the busy schedule of hospitals and especially of emergency departments, some patients are indeed neglected. A seriously ill child may not be recognized as such by a receptionist or nurse or may not be brought to the doctor's attention for treatment. A physician's own busyness, tiredness or lack of experience may result in inadequate or inappropriate treatment. A child with a severe illness may be sent home after emergency treatment when, in fact, he should have been admitted to the hospital. Occasionally, some children with a chronic illness are labeled "chronic complainers." This may lead to genuine complaints of being ignored and untreated.

The complex process of delivering medical care in hospitals is not understood by the public and produces many situations which can be interpreted by parents as instances of neglect or inadequate or improper treatment. Such complexity may also arouse severe anger and violence in some predisposed individuals.

Miscommunication

Miscommunication may occur on both verbal and nonverbal levels. For example, verbal instructions given to a patient may be negated by the physician's nonverbal attitude, which indicates to the patient that the doctor does not believe the treatment prescribed will make much difference in the outcome of the patient's disease or which indicates that the physician was prescribing medication just to get rid of the patient. The noncompliance of patients often results from contradictory messages of this sort.

Lack of clear instructions adds to the patient's confusion and leads to miscommunication. Physician's orders, when not expressed clearly or when not clearly written, may be misinterpreted by the nurse and miscommunicated to the patient. These problems in communication may lead to inappropriate or inadequate management of the child and, consequently, contribute to the parent's anger.

Misunderstanding

Misunderstandings are also frequently based on miscommunication, though the parents' own personality difficulties, preconceived ideas and expectations may contribute to the misinterpretation of clearly given verbal instructions.

How to Handle Irate Parents

Don't Display Anger

Some physicians feel quite angry at the irate parents and would like to kick them out of the hospital or eject them from their office (Lion, 1973). But if treatment is to continue, this anger must not be exhibited. Keeping in mind the multitude of reasons for the parents' anger, the physician's overt reaction of anger without investigation into and understanding of the causes of the parents' anger would itself be irrational and unjustified. Moreover, once the physician's anger is overtly displayed, he quickly loses control of the situation. His overt expression of anger can only serve to generate more anxiety in himself, in the nursing staff and in nearby patients. The best the physician can do in these situations is to minimize the disruption (Schulman, 1970).

First, get the child of irate parents out of the waiting or triage area as soon as a room is available. Then either have the child wait his turn or see him as quickly as possible, perhaps before other patients with minor illnesses. If the irate parents respond to these calming measures—such as seeing the patient briefly and ordering any necessary laboratory work—the physician has more time. But if the belligerent attitude of the parents persists, the physician is probably better off seeing their child ahead of turn. The longer irate parents are around, the more confusion and disruption there is likely to be.

This approach—prompt treatment and release—is applicable to children with whom you anticipate only brief contact, not to those you expect to treat and follow over a long period of time. In the latter case, this approach may serve only to reinforce the irate behavior of the parents. The anger of these parents needs to be dealt with in an interview situation.

Another precaution is to carefully document the examination and treatment of these patients. While this should always be the case, it is particularly important with parents who have personality problems. Be sure to include in the chart all your recommendations and instructions to the child and to the parents, along with a note indicating that you have discussed possible side effects of prescribed medication.

Be Aware of Parental Personality Problems

People with an aggressive personality style react to mild frustrations with aggressive outbursts. Individuals with a hysterical personality style may exaggerate various aspects of their child's illness. Persons with an antisocial personality may lie and may distort the situation to their benefit. These parental personality problems are not likely to respond to one session of counseling. The physician may be getting into serious difficulty if he tries to use "I'll teach them" type tactics. Many of these people do not learn from one experience, and it may only serve to accentuate their personality characteristics.

Avoid the Risk of Assault

Assault on hospital staff is not an uncommon occurrence and is certainly on the increase. There is, however, little consensus and few guidelines about dealing with adults who become enraged and behave in a threatening and violent manner. Acute and frequently unexpected episodes of assault result in injuries to these adults as well as to persons around them and cause disruption of treatment programs. Furthermore, the legal complications arising from attempts to deal with such episodes are difficult to resolve and are characterized by much adverse publicity.

If the rage of an adult appears to have reached a point where assault appears imminent and further talking is not likely to calm the person down, it is important to call the security guard or police officer for assistance. Delay can only disrupt the situation further.

Dealing directly with violent individuals requires a great deal of experience and understanding. Frazier (1977) feels that "talking is the best way to neutralize a violent patient—even when he carries a weapon." Noting the difficulty of appearing unafraid when facing an unremorseful murderer with a gun, he reported having said on such an occasion, "I don't feel comfortable with you pointing that loaded gun at me. Why don't you put it down?" He emphasized that the last thing one does with a disturbed, violent person is struggle. He characterized a disturbed, violent individual as a "loner, a social isolate, a battered child, parentless or without a father, who has not learned to handle aggression." Such individuals never had the opportunity of telling anyone of their frustrations, fears and failures. Once they realize that someone is going to listen to them, they may calm down.

Interview

When angry parents are available for an interview, they should be seen as soon as possible in a quiet office setting. Such an interview should never be carried out in the patient waiting area or in corridors in a hurried fashion. The following points will help facilitate a good interview:

ALLOW VENTILATION.—It is important to listen to the accumulated complaints of long-standing duration or to acute problems of recent origin. A keen listening posture on the part of the interviewer will promote ventilation of such problems. A nod of the head or a positive verbal comment such as, "I am beginning to understand why you feel this way," or "Please go on," will encourage individuals to continue talking about their problems.

OBSERVE BODILY EXPRESSIONS.—As the interview progresses, observing physical manifestations of tension, anger and relaxation helps the physician to gauge the effects of the interview. An acutely angry individual looks tense, has a rigid posture and a flushed face, may be breathing faster than normal and may sit at the edge of the chair. Success of the interview is reflected by the disappearance of anger from the face, relaxation of posture and reduction of tension. This usually occurs after the individual has verbalized sufficiently about his gripes so that he is willing to assess the situation more objectively.

Occasionally, one comes across angry parents who seem to have made up their mind about the situation and have rationalized their anger. They are not willing to talk about the problem and do not respond to talking. Their anger is frequently based on long-term difficulties with physicians and hospitals. Many of these cases end up in court as malpractice suits.

DETERMINE THE CAUSE OF ANGER.—Factors which contribute to and precipitate anger in the parents are multiple, and it is not always possible to determine the exact cause of the anger. Frequently, several external factors interacting with personality problems precipitate the anger. Personal and family difficulties may complicate the issue and lower the individual's threshold for becoming angry. It is not necessary, however, to determine the exact cause of anger in order to resolve the problem. It may be sufficient to define a general area or source of difficulty.

DETERMINE WHAT THE INTERVIEWEE WANTS.—One of the most important aspects of the interview, besides promotion of ventilation, is to determine what the interviewee wants. Anger is an emotion that is triggered when a human being faces a situation that requires fighting back. If the anger is aroused by a multitude of factors, it is generally diffuse. Simple ventilation will help dissipate anger. Most of these parents may not want anything more than to express their anger and to be satisfied that their point of view has been heard.

When anger is directed toward a specific target, such as a person or a group of persons, it is not easily dissipated without being inflicted upon the target in some manner. Shouting, name calling and hitting affect the target and help dissipate the anger. Certainly, the degree of vengeance felt by different individuals varies. Some people may be satisfied with the correction of the situation and the consequently better treatment of their child. Others may demand that the person responsible for their difficulties be in some way admonished.

The interviewer should ask the parents for their suggestions for correcting the problem. Most parents respond to such questions with broad comments, e.g., "We don't want this situation to be repeated," "We don't want other people to go through the same thing," or "We think this person should be talked to or transferred to another part of the hospital where he will not have to deal with people." Since the majority of people are not familiar with the complexity of hospital functions, they rarely offer more specific suggestions.

ADMISSION OF MISTAKES.—If the interviewer is not part of the problem, he should not admit to the mistakes of other personnel. He should limit himself instead to making general comments, such as, "We try to teach all our personnel to provide the best medical care, but we are not always successful," or "There are many people who are not as courteous as others."

TERMINATION.—The interviewer should outline a specific plan of action before termination of the interview. The plan may be quite specific or very general, depending upon the cause of the problem and the demands of the parents. The interviewer should promise the parents that he will keep them informed on how the plan of action is progressing and on the outcomes achieved.

REFERENCES

Frazier, S. H.: Talking is the best way to neutralize the violent patient, Roche Report, September 15, 1977, p. 3.

Lion, J. R., and Pasternak, S. A.: Counter-transference reaction to violent patients, Am. J. Psychiatry 130:207, 1973.

Schulman, J. L.: The management of the irate parent, J. Pediatr. 77:338, 1970.

15/Psychiatric Interviews with Parents and Children

INTERVIEWING IS AN ART that requires much practice before it is mastered. The interview is a tool that allows a physician or psychiatrist to transmit and apply his special knowledge. Through the interview, the physician gathers data that help him understand the problem of his patient. Although the interviewer is usually perceived as an authority figure who asks the questions and directs the interview, the interview may best be conceptualized as a form of communication between the interviewer and his patient.

The first interview usually takes place between strangers—the doctor and his patient never having seen each other before. This situation normally arouses some anxiety, even in the most experienced interviewer. It is important for the interviewer to recognize his own feelings of anxiety, as this will help him empathize with the anxiety of his patient. The first interview is not simply a friendly conversation with a stranger. The patient comes with certain expectations and is required to reveal a great deal of himself before the interviewer can help him. Revealing oneself is a very difficult task, even for a needy patient. There are many psychological processes that obstruct free communication between the interviewer and the patient, the most common of these processes being transference, resistance and countertransference.

Transference

Transference is a psychological process whereby the patient unconsciously and inappropriately displaces and projects onto individuals in his current life those patterns of behavior and emotional reactions associated with the significant figures of his childhood. The patient's previous relationships with other persons influence his present relationship with the interviewer. His relationship with his parents may have particular importance because it is the first and often the strongest of the patient's relationships. If the patient had and continues to have a constructive and friendly relationship with his father, it should facilitate the development of a friendly relationship with a male interviewer. If his father was or is harsh and punitive, on the other hand, the patient may expect the interviewer to be critical of him. Similarly, previous experiences with other physicians or psychiatrists are likely to influence, at least initially, the present relationship with the interviewer.

The external and explicit features of the interviewer may serve as the starting point of transference. The interviewer's age, sex, personality, mannerisms, social and ethnic background—all influence the rapidity and direction of transference. An older female patient may, for example, treat a young male interviewer as her son and be very helpful and supportive. The nature and intensity of the illness may also influence the needs of the patient and the development of transference.

Infantile feelings of parental omnipotence or of rebelliousness are frequently directed toward the interviewer, who may have trouble understanding such inappropriate reactions. In his perplexity, the interviewer may feel that his own behavior has been seriously amiss, or he may become angry at the patient.

The term "positive transference" is often employed to refer to all of the patient's positive responses to the interviewer. However, the patient's realistic and appropriate responses to the interviewer are not transference.

Recognition of transference is the most important first step in dealing with it. The patient who trusts the interviewer is easier to work with than the patient who is constantly doubting and questioning him. Positive transference does not need to be interpreted in the initial sessions. In fact, the interviewer may take advantage of the patient's positive feelings toward him to develop a more realistic, positive relationship. A patient's rebellious and negative attitude toward the interviewer interferes with therapeutic progress and hinders the development of a working relationship with the interviewer. This attitude, if based on transference, should be brought up for discussion after the first few sessions. One should not, however, interpret the transference at this early stage by saying, for example, "You are angry at me because you had similar feelings toward your father." The negative attitude needs to be worked through over a period of several sessions. The interviewer may begin by pointing out the angry, sullen or negative affect of the patient: "You look very angry," or "You sounded very negative when you talked about . . . ." The interviewer should explore the underlying reasons for this affect. Initially, the patient may give explanations that are only tangentially related to his anger. The intensity of the negative affect, however, indicates that the patient is not aware of the real reasons, especially those deriving from and based upon childhood relationships. Insight into transference reactions is acquired only gradually, over a long period of time.

Resistance

Resistance is any attitude on the part of the patient that opposes the objectives of the treatment. Resistance may stem from various sources, such as repression (an attempt to ward off threatening impulses by keeping them out of awareness), transference, the need to maintain the secondary gain of the illness or a punitive superego demanding punishment (as in depression).

Resistance is frequently manifested in the interview by silence or by the patient's declaring, "I don't have anything to talk about today." Ignoring the interviewer's question or abruptly changing the subject under discussion may also indicate resistance. Some patients express resistance through intellectualization and verboseness. Generalizing rather than focusing specifically on himself, changing appointment times and coming late for appointments also reflect varying degrees of resistance.

Countertransference

The interviewer's attitude has an important influence on his relationship with his patients. He should try to become aware of his thoughts, feelings, strengths and shortcomings. Some patients arouse certain thoughts and feelings which give the interviewer further clues to his attitude. By becoming more aware of his reactions to his patient, the interviewer can become more effective in controlling his inappropriate responses. For instance, his awareness that certain patients make him feel angry, discouraged or irritated may help the interviewer curtail the display of these feelings.

Most interviewers identify with their patients to a greater or lesser degree. If he dislikes his patient, the interviewer is prone to be ineffective in dealing with him. If the interviewer is hostile, the patient becomes more hostile, leading to a rapid deterioration of the relationship. If the interviewer feels antagonism, he should try to evaluate the basis for this feeling. There is a bit of the howling, enraged child in most patients, even in good ones who are usually defined as cooperative. It is the patient's childish, hostile and demanding attitude that the interviewer must learn to deal with effectively to avoid development of countertransference.

Countertransference may be manifested by overidentification with the patient. The interviewer who overidentifies with his patient may have difficulty recognizing or understanding problems similar to his own. Power struggles, arguing with, competing with or badgering the patient are familiar examples of countertransference. With older patients, countertransference may be manifested by the wish to be the patient's child or younger sibling.

Who Should Be Interviewed First?

Children rarely come to see a psychiatrist of their own free will. They are brought by their parents or other adults who become concerned about some aspect of their behavior. Children frequently locate the causes of their difficulties in their environment. If a child is not doing well in school, he is likely to attribute this to the meanness of his teacher or to other children distracting him. If he has difficulty in getting along with peers or siblings, he feels that it is his peers or siblings who are at fault. It is only through repeated support and assurance that a child begins to discriminate between his own contribution and the contribution of others to his problems.

In pediatric practice, parents provide a major part of the medical and psychiatric history. Learning to deal with parents is thus as important as learning to interview children. When a child is brought by his parents, the question arises of who should be seen first, the child, the parents or the parents and the child together? Clinicians vary in their approach to the first interview depending upon their experience, training and time constraints. Some interviewers prefer seeing the parents and the child together, while others see them in separate sessions. Including the child in the first session with the parents has some disadvantages: most parents are uncomfortable and reluctant to talk about the problems of their child in the child's presence, and they often avoid talking about themselves as well. Proponents of the family interview, however, argue that the roots of the problem are frequently the isolation of the child and lack of openness in family communication. Seeing parents and child separately only promotes the isolation and secretiveness that characterize problem families and creates doubt in the mind of the child about the clinician's ability to help him. There are few parents, however, who are willing to discuss the problems of the family in the presence of the child. A young child is also likely to misinterpret and misunderstand some of the problems his parents discuss in the family session. In general, then, it is much more comfortable for the parents if they are interviewed separately from the child in the initial diagnostic session.

Different types of interviews are best suited for obtaining specific types of information. For example, a family interview offers an opportunity to observe the interaction among the various members of the family, while a group interview with peers is more revealing of problems of social interaction. An interview should be planned on the basis of the type of information that the physician wants to obtain for diagnostic purposes. In psychiatric work with children, different types of interviews are scheduled at different times to obtain specific information on various facets of the child's life. For instance, parents are seen first in order to obtain information about their perception of the child's problem, as well as for information about marital and other problems between the parents. The child is interviewed alone to hear his side of the story and to observe his behavior, especially in relation to the interviewer. The child is seen with the parents or with the rest of the family to observe the family's interaction. The child may also need to be observed with a group of children, such as in the classroom, on a playground or in a therapy group of children.

Diagnostic Interview with Parents

Most parents are very anxious during the first interview. Many of them feel guilty and responsible for their child's problems. Some parents fear that the clinician will blame them for having caused their child's problems. For these reasons, parents are very defensive and guarded, especially during the first interview. Generally, fathers are more defensive than mothers. It may be because most fathers have less experience dealing with clinicians than do mothers, or it may be because most fathers spend very little time with their children and feel guilty and more responsible when their children have problems. Clinicians should insist on seeing both parents in intact families during the first interview. Pediatricians are used to seeing mothers with the children and frequently feel uncomfortable in the presence of fathers. In our experience, the father's absence from the first interview may be the result of the clinician's own avoidance or the mother's attempt to keep her husband out of the picture. Direct communication with the father usually increases the probability of his attendance.

The interviewer must help the anxious parents to feel relaxed and less defensive. The interviewer can do this by maintaining a respectful attitude toward the parents and by talking about a neutral subject for a few minutes (e.g., difficulties in taking time off to come for the interview). The interviewer need not worry about starting the interview, as most parents have a lot on their minds and will begin talking about their problem without prompting. If there is silence, the interviewer can get the parents started by asking them about their current problems with the child. It is extremely important to allow the parents to follow their own associations in describing their problems, at least during the first half of the interview. In other words, let the parents talk without interruption. Make a mental note of what the parents emphasize and what aspects of the problem they avoid. There is usually a pause after parents have given their version of the problem. The pause frequently indicates that the parents want some direction as to how to proceed further. At this time, the interviewer may inquire about the aspects of the problem that have been neglected. He should avoid, however, exploring areas on which parents seem touchy. Remember that for many parents this may be their first contact with the helping or psychiatric profession. A child with severe or moderate emotional problems is likely to need psychiatric services for quite some time. Early probing into sensitive areas is likely to drive many parents away from seeking further or sustained psychiatric help.

The initial interview with parents who have already been seen by some other clinician or in some other agency differs somewhat in content, although the goal of the interview remains the same as described above. The interviewer may indicate that he has already talked with the referring clinician or agency or has read the report sent by them but would like to hear more details directly from the parents. Later, he should also explore the understanding of the problem that the parents have derived from other clinicians or agencies.

Some parents come to an interview unwillingly, on orders from a school, a court or a social agency. They come unwillingly because they do not consider their child to be a problem. They project blame onto the school, the teachers, the social agency or society at large. They are extremely defensive and angry and may regard the interviewer as part of the same harmful system and direct some of their anger toward him. The interviewer should listen to their story with genuine interest. Although he may not agree with their perception of the problem, he should save his questions for later, since premature questioning drives these parents away from further involvement with the clinician. The ultimate goal of helping these parents—and the child—is achieved only with continuous support from the interviewer over a prolonged period of time.

Later Interviews

The plan of treatment should be laid out during the first interview, and the hour and date should be set for the second interview. During later interviews, further exploration of the child's problems is made in the context of his family and peer relationships. Detailed information is gathered about the onset of the problem, the child's developmental history, family history, medical history, school achievement and peer relationships. Although some guidance is necessary, the parents should be allowed to describe the events and problems in their own words. The interviewer should also make a note of the affect associated with the content, since observation of affect frequently provides clues to areas of resistance and repression. The interviewer may, for example, begin to suspect repression of affect if a parent expresses little emotion while describing the death of a sibling or when parents avoid discussing marital problems despite the interviewer's questions about such problems.

It is important to develop a working relationship with the parents. The parents should regard the diagnostic process as a collaborative effort on the part of the interviewer and themselves and should be encouraged to explore all factors contributing to the child's problems. This type of cooperation is not always easy to achieve, especially with parents who are unwilling participants or who are hostile toward the helping professionals. Creating an atmosphere of openness and honesty and clearly stating the goals of the interview will promote the development of a good working relationship. As there are many facets to the diagnostic work-up that may appear irrelevant to the parents, it is helpful to state and clarify the purpose of every aspect of the work-up in order to obtain their full cooperation. For example, most parents do not comprehend the relationship between their marital problems and their child's behavioral problems. The interviewer must explain to the parents that the child is an integral part of the family and that he is influenced by all aspects of family relationships, including the dissatisfaction and resentment experienced in the marital relationship.

Asking evocative questions is basic to the ongoing process of the interview, since it stimulates and encourages the parents to explore new problem areas. When the interviewer asks a question, he brings into the open the feelings connected with the question and prepares parents for greater understanding. Open-ended questions are good elicitors of information. Questions of "why" frequently lead to an intellectual response. More emotionally evocative questions usually relate to the "how," "when," "where" or "what" of the events. For example, one may ask the parents, "Could you explain this further?" "How did this happen?" "What do you mean?"

There are many aspects of the family relationship that may be quite embarrassing for the parents, as well as for the interviewer, to discuss openly. Discussion of finances, family secrets, sexual practices and sexual problems may be very sensitive topics for many parents. The inexperienced interviewer usually avoids exploring these areas, either by denying their relevance to the child's problems or by asking questions in a manner that promotes further denial. For instance, such direct questioning as, "Do you have any problems in your sexual relationship?" frequently draws a negative reply. The interviewer should reserve the exploration of sensitive areas for later interviews and should discuss them in the context of the parents' relationship with each other, starting with, "How do you get along with each other?" "How do you feel toward each other?" and, exploring further, "How do you feel about your sexual relationship?" "Are there questions in this area that you may have but have not discussed with each other?"

Family secrets also create problems and confusion for the children. Some children may avoid talking to anyone about anything because they have been forbidden to talk about some family secret. The parents themselves may keep secrets from each other, such as extramarital relations or financial arrangments. Such secrets create doubt, suspicion and a lack of open communication between the parents.

Some parents ask the interviewer for guidance and advice before he is able to gather the information necessary to give such advice. The interviewer should refrain from offering premature advice based on insufficient data or from giving his opinions on spiritual or moral issues. While the intent may be to help the parents, such opinions frequently convey the counselor's biases to them. In addition, these opinions may lead the parents to perceive the counselor as an omniscient, preaching or paternalistic figure, which perception will prevent them from developing a working relationship with him.

Special Types of Interviews

Many modes and styles of interviews have evolved from different theoretical backgrounds or have been developed to meet the special needs of patients.

NONDIRECTIVE INTERVIEWS.—In this type of interview, the interviewer remains nondirective throughout the interview. He listens to his patients with interest and repeats the last word or the last sentence of the patient to promote further verbalization during a pause. This approach is based on the theory that the patient possesses all the necessary information and abilities to resolve his problems and that sooner or later he will unearth the curative information or abilities if he can simply talk about his problems to an interested passive listener.

INTERVIEWS WITH ANXIOUS PATIENTS.—Here, the interviewer should make a special attempt to reduce the anxiety of his overanxious patients by relaxing himself, by talking about neutral subjects for a few minutes and even by asking the patient if he can do anything to make the patient more comfortable. Most patients begin to relax by the second or third interview, so that their anxiety is then related to the stress of the interview rather than the process of being interviewed per se. Patients who remain anxious even after several interviews probably suffer from chronic anxiety, which is aggravated by any type of minor stress.

CONSULTATION INTERVIEWS.—Many consultations in medicine are consultee-oriented, that is, they relate to the specific questions of the physician requesting the consultation with regard to the patient's diagnosis, prognosis or treatment.

Requests for psychiatric consultation are, however, frequently ambiguous. It is a mistake to plunge into a consultation without clarifying the matters to be discussed with the consultee. Preferably, the consultant should talk to the consultee directly to clarify what is desired from the consultation, and the consultant should be sure that the consultee has already informed the patient about the psychiatric consultation. The consultation interview is a standard diagnostic interview in which, however, the consultant is much more active and directive. There is frequently a tendency on the part of the psychiatric consultant to form quick impressions on the basis of insufficient data. Such tendencies should be avoided. The psychiatric consultant is not always able to answer all the consultee's questions in a single brief interview. Some questions require a complete diagnostic work-up before they can be answered satisfactorily. It is the responsibility of the consultee to inform his patient of the findings of the psychiatric consultation, but he may ask the psychiatric consultant to assist him in explaining the findings.

BEHAVIORAL INTERVIEW.—The content of the behavioral interview may be quite different from that of a traditional interview. The primary function of the behavioral interview is to obtain descriptive information about the child's problem behavior and the conditions that maintain it. The interviewer does not explore the family dynamics or developmental history.

Diagnostic Interviews with Children

Young children are frequently anxious and unhappy about visiting a physician. Their anxiety is usually related to being in a strange place, meeting a strange person, sharing some of the parents' anxiety and having fearful fantasies about the visit. Previsit preparation by the parents may lessen some of the child's anxiety. At the time when the parents make an appointment for the child, the psychiatrist should tell the parents how to prepare their child for his visit. The parents should be advised to explain the purpose of the visit to the child in a plain and simple manner. The visit to the psychiatrist should be distinguished from other visits to physicians when the child received injections and medications. The purpose of the visit may be verbalized as, "We want you to talk with Dr. Smith about your stomach pains. We think that perhaps you have these pains because you don't feel good about something," or "We all want to talk with Dr. Smith to find out why we don't get along well with each other." There should be no connotation of punishment in the parents' explanation of the visit. With older children and when parents have already been interviewed by the psychiatrist, the parents may tell the child that they have already talked with the psychiatrist about how they feel about the problem, and now the psychiatrist wants to talk with the child about how he feels about the situation.

The psychiatrist should try to observe the child with his parents before meeting him. The child's manner of relating to his parents in the waiting room may not be typical of his usual relationship with them, but it may be indicative of his behavior in stressful situations. The psychiatrist should converse with the parents for a few minutes and allow them to introduce the child to him. When greeting the child, the psychiatrist should bend down to the level of the child's eyes while shaking his hand and avoid changing his voice to a childish or singsong tone while talking to the child. He should explain to the child that he wants to talk with him alone in his office, which is located nearby. Then the psychiatrist should ask the parents to wait there until he and the child are finished talking.

In most cases, the psychiatrist does not encounter any difficulty in bringing the child to his office. However, some frightened younger children may hang on to their parents and refuse to leave them. It serves no therapeutic purpose to separate the child forcibly from his parents. In such cases, the psychiatrist should sit down with the family and talk to them for a few minutes, explaining to them the purpose of the visit—that he wants to talk with the child and that there are some toys in his office that the child can play with and that there will not be any injections. If the child continues to be reluctant to accompany him, the psychiatrist should invite the parents to go with the child to his office. In the office, the psychiatrist should allow the child to explore the office or to play with some toys. He should look for an opportunity when the young child will be willing to play with him or to draw a picture with him. Once the child begins to relax, the psychiatrist may ask the child if it is all right for his parents to wait outside in the waiting room. If the child's anxiety does not diminish and he continues hanging on to his parents, the psychiatrist should conduct the interview as a family interview. It sometimes takes several family sessions before the child is able to separate from his parents, which produces a great deal of anxiety in both the parents and the psychiatrist. Anxiety and awkwardness can be avoided if the separation problem is anticipated in advance of the first interview with the parents. The parents may be told that in case of separation difficulty, a family interview will be conducted.

After a few minutes of conversation on such neutral topics as where the child lives and goes to school and whether he has siblings, the initial part of the interview with the child involves helping him understand the purpose of the visit and allaying his anxiety and fears about the visit.

The psychiatrist should ask the child about the purpose of the visit—his own understanding and whatever his parents might have told him about it. The psychiatrist may then ask the child if he knows what kind of doctor the psychiatrist is and what psychiatrists do with children who visit them. If the child expresses his ignorance, the psychiatrist should explain, "I am a doctor who talks with children. I talk with children who may have difficulty in getting along with their parents, with their brothers and sisters, with their friends. . . ." "I also like to help children who do not like school, who get into fights with other children, or have temper tantrums. . . ." The psychiatrist should deliver this explanation very slowly, with frequent pauses to give the child a chance to think or make comments. Some children respond by picking out one of the problems mentioned by the psychiatrist, such as a child who says, "Yes, I don't like to go to school," or "I hate school." Such verbalizations facilitate further exploration of the problem. The most important goal of the initial interview with the child is to develop an alliance with him so that he can feel relaxed and begin to express his thoughts and feelings.

The purpose of the interview with the child is to make a clinical assessment of his personality, emotional status, mental capacity and general functioning. The psychiatrist evaluates these things by observing and communicating with the child. The communication, however, should be appropriate to the child's age and level of intellectual functioning. Young children communicate easily through their play. A standard set of toys—a rubber doll family, a wooden house or school, a toy telephone, a styrofoam ball, some clay, crayons and paper—is used in this type of communication.

Young children's play can be structured by setting up a situation with the doll family, in which the child doll is expected to interact with other members of the family. A great deal of information may be elicited about the child's feelings and fantasies through structured and unstructured play. Verbal communication obviously aids enormously in understanding the child and should be used as much as possible.

Most school-age children are able to sit and talk for only short periods of time and soon become uncomfortable with this adult mode of communication. Some psychiatrists utilize a combined technique of communication through conversation and dialogue during play. For instance, during structured play with dolls, the psychiatrist can orchestrate a dialogue among different members of the family. A basic assumption in this situation is that the child identifies with the child doll of his or her sex and that all the thoughts and feelings expressed by the child doll reflect the child's own thoughts and feelings. Almost any type of medium—clay, drawings, puppets, drama, painting—that children are accustomed to in play activities can be utilized during interviews to communicate with the child.

Children's drawings reveal a great deal about them. They may be asked to draw a person, themselves and their family. The drawing of the family may be a kinetic drawing in which every member is doing something. Such drawings reveal the family's style of living and the way various members interact with one another. Drawings are also used to assess the overall intellectual potential of the child and serve as projections of the child's feelings and fantasies. The psychiatrist may ask the child to make up a story about his drawing. The story-making process can be helped along by the psychiatrist asking questions about the beginning, middle and end of the story. Drawings of a house or a school can be used to understand the child's relationship with the occupants of the house or school, such as teacher and peers.

The termination of the interview should be signaled in advance to give the child enough time to pick up the toys and tidy the playroom. The psychiatrist, being an equal partner in the play, should assist in the cleanup. Children should not be allowed to break or destroy toys or other objects in the office or the playroom. Such destructive acts make children feel guilty and unhappy.

Mental Status Examination of a Child

The report of the mental status examination of a child includes much of the same information that is elicited by a standard psychiatric examination: the child's general appearance, physique, relationship with parents and examiner, dominant affect, ability to converse, thought content, understanding of the problem, an overall assessment of intellectual potential, the presence of obvious physical abnormality and the level of general motor coordination. It is difficult to determine the presence of delusion and hallucinations in young children, as their verbalizations normally contain many fantasies. However, most children are able to differentiate fantasies from realities.

Interviews with Adolescents

Interviews with adolescents require special preparation. Adolescents aspire to being treated like adults and resent it if their parents force them to see a psychiatrist. In order to minimize the negative reaction of the adolescent to the psychiatrist, some preparation of the adolescent is essential prior to the first interview. If the adolescent is willing to see a psychiatrist, he should preferably be seen first during the initial visit, ahead of the parents. This gesture is usually interpreted by the adolescent to mean that the psychiatrist gives him primary importance and is more interested in him than in his parents. Many adolescents have suspicious and negative feelings toward the psychiatrist if their parents are interviewed first—their meeting being interpreted as the adults (parents and the psychiatrist) plotting together against the adolescent. They are generally very observant of any evidence of insincerity in adults.

When an adolescent is unwilling to see a psychiatrist, a great deal of preliminary counseling with the parents may be necessary to help them motivate the adolescent to enter psychotherapy. The parents are seen in several sessions designed to help them understand the nature of their relationship with and the problems of their adolescent. The parents are asked to share the understanding they have achieved through counseling with their adolescent. They may say, "We found talking to the psychiatrist very helpful. However, he is very interested in talking with you and wants to hear your side of the story." Some of these resistant adolescents will refuse to be interviewed alone but may agree to be seen with their family. It is quite common for the adolescent to be belligerent and uncommunicative, and the psychiatrist should respect the adolescent's right to behave in this manner.

Individual sessions with depressed adolescents are very challenging for the psychiatrist. Such sessions require the active participation of the psychiatrist. A depressed adolescent wants the psychiatrist to take care of him. The very nature of the depression makes him pessimistic about the outcome of the condition and causes him to withdraw from his environment. The depressed adolescent lacks spontaneity and may stare blankly into space or down at the floor. Structuring the interview to discuss various aspects of daily life may make the interview more productive. Comments about the adolescent's depressed mood may elicit some response from the patient. A depressed, withdrawn youngster does not become emotionally engaged with the interviewer. Suicidal risk should be evaluated in every depressed adolescent, and hospitalization may be required for further management.

Diagnostic Family Session Interview

A diagnostic family interview offers an excellent opportunity for the psychiatrist to observe the patterns of interaction among various members of the family and to understand the family dynamics that influence the problem child. It is important to have all the members of the family at this interview, including any babies. Most parents find it difficult to comprehend the need for a family session interview. Since the parents provide most of the diagnostic information about the child's development and his interaction with other members of the family, they may interpret the psychiatrist's desire to interview the whole family as an expression of his lack of trust in them or in their ability to provide reliable information.

Some parents are reluctant to bring their family to the interview because they have not told the siblings about the patient. In one such case, the parents explained that they did not want to tell the siblings because they were likely to share the information with their friends, who would then tease the patient about being "crazy."

Some parents fear that the family session may have a traumatic impact on the younger sibling(s). Talking about an 8-year-old sibling, one parent remarked, "She would not understand. She is just a little innocent child. She wouldn't know what this is all about." The reluctance of parents to accept the need for a family session interview frequently arises from lack of open communication within the family. Different members of such families keep secrets from one another. Getting together in a family session may imply that everybody will be exposed and that their secrets will no longer remain secret. The other children in such families offer as much resistance to coming for a family session interview as do the parents. All kinds of excuses are made to avoid attending the family session interview. In fact, one often finds that the members of such a family rarely ever get together for anything.

The psychiatrist should explain to the parents that the family session interview is part of the routine diagnostic process and is designed to help the psychiatrist understand the relationships among various members of the family. He should explore the concerns and the feelings of the parents about the family session interview. He should emphasize strongly that during the family session interview he will not divulge any information about any family member that was derived from a prior individual interview with that individual. The psychiatrist may, however, tell the parents that, in his experience, children already know about most of the family secrets. Due to lack of complete information and to secrecy in the family, children are forced to fill in the blanks with their own imaginings. Moreover, efforts to hide certain family matters from children place a great burden on the parents and may be interpreted by the children as evidence of parental rejection.

Some preparation of siblings at home before the family session interview is extremely helpful in assuring a successful interview. The psychiatrist should suggest that parents call a family meeting at home and explain to all siblings the purpose of the family session interview with the psychiatrist. The parents may say, "Johnny has some difficulty in getting along in school. We have talked with a psychiatrist to find out how best to help Johnny. The psychiatrist wants to meet the whole family to find out how we get along and how we can all best help Johnny." Questions from siblings should be answered honestly and simply. They may be told to act naturally in the psychiatrist's office and to talk about whatever they like without censoring their remarks out of fear of parental reprisal.

Families in a psychiatrist's office show different patterns of conflict and anxiety. Typically, the family arrives in a state of tension and apprehension. The children are quiet, reserved and on their best behavior. The parents or the psychiatrist may reduce the anxiety by talking about the problem. Each child may be asked to express his perception of the problem.

Family therapists frequently regard the family as a functioning unit and consider the problems of the individual members as the result of some basic underlying problem(s) in the family system. Although different family members, by virtue of different physical and mental capacities, may express the problem differently, they are regarded as reacting to the same basic problem. Thus, after anxiety is reduced and communication has improved, the psychiatrist tries to find a basic problem in the family system. Various types of family systems and family interaction have been described that lead to problems in individual members of the family.

Some families put up a good front as if nothing is wrong—no one in the family is allowed to criticize or talk negatively about other family members. At the other end of the spectrum, there are families in which nobody agrees on anything, and there is constant bickering and arguing over every matter. Recognition of the various patterns of family functioning is helpful in both the diagnosis and the planning of family treatment.

ADDITIONAL READING

Edinburg, G. M., Linberg, N. E., and Kelman, W.: *Clinical Interviewing and Counseling: Principles and Techniques* (New York: Appleton-Century-Crofts, 1975).

Lewin, K.: Behavior and Development as a Function of the Total Situation, in Carmichael, L. (ed.): *Manual of Child Psychology* (New York: John Wiley, 1946, pp. 791–844).

Mackinnon, R. A., and Michels, R.: *The Psychiatric Interview in Clinical Practice* (Philadelphia: W. B. Saunders Co., 1971).

Stevenson, I.: *Medical History Taking* (New York: Hoeber, Inc., 1960).

16/Basic Issues in Malpractice

INADVERTENT INVOLVEMENT in malpractice suits is a constant concern for most physicians and other health care personnel. Emergency care settings are especially likely to involve medical personnel in such suits. This chapter describes the basic issues in malpractice that every health care professional should become familiar with and it also offers some suggestions to strengthen the doctor-patient relationship so as to minimize the occurrence of malpractice suits.

The word "malpractice" denotes fault or bad practice. When a person is injured by medical treatment, he is ordinarily not entitled to compensation unless he can prove that his injury was caused by a negligent act of omission on the part of a member of a health care team. In broad terms, "medical injury" is a disability caused by medical management. The term "medical management" includes both actions taken and failures to act, but it does not imply that the management was necessarily improper.

Disability, in a broad sense, means to be deprived of normal functioning. In a medical injury context, disability takes many forms, including physical and mental impairment, disfigurement and pain and suffering. Often, several forms are present in a single injury.

Medical injuries can result from physician error but can also occur in the absence of such error. An illustrative example is a comparison of 2 patients, each of whom experienced a disabling allergic reaction to a penicillin injection. One patient had taken penicillin on prior occasions without experiencing any adverse effects. The other patient had suffered shortness of breath and skin rash after a previous use of penicillin, and the injection notation ALLERGIC PENICILLIN appeared in large prominent letters on the jacket of his medical record. Both patients contracted streptococcal pharyngitis. Their physicians ordered a penicillin injection, and both patients suffered disabling reactions. In the first case, the physician made no error, and yet the patient suffered a medical injury because it was the treatment and not the disease which caused his disability. In the second case, the physician was negligent in that he knew, or should have known, that his patient was allergic to penicillin. He could have prevented the allergic reaction by giving some other appropriate drug. In this example, both patients suffered medical injury, but negligence was a factor in only one of them.

Scope of the Problem

The report of the HEW Secretary's Commission on Medical Malpractice (1973) indicated that an estimated 12,000 incidents triggered malpractice claim file action reaching settlement in 1970, approximately one third of which were warning files rather than true claims. About 40% of the true incidents eventuated in payments to claimants. The total compensation to claimants was estimated to be $80,300,000. The median payment was $2,000. Payments varied widely in amount, however, with a noticeable number being in the $5,000 to $8,000 range and one half of the payments being in amounts of less than $2,000. Payment in excess of $100,000 were infrequent (3%), but they contributed substantially to the aggregate cost.

The injuries alleged to be iatrogenic occurred when patients were being treated for a variety of ailments. Orthopedic surgery, gastrointestinal surgery and gynecologic treatment generated the largest number of malpractice suits. The type of negligence claimed as resulting in injury was predominantly that of improper treatment (86%), as opposed to failure to diagnose properly. Malpractice incidents usually occurred in hospital settings (75%), such as the surgical suite (39%) or the patient's room (34%). Emergency room and intensive care facilities accounted for only 13% of such incidents.

The report also categorized the injuries by severity. The majority of the injuries sustained were found to be minor and temporary (50.9%), with little or no delay in recovery. However, sizable numbers of incidents involved more severe injury or fatality (20.8%). Severity of injury was systematically related to the ultimate disposition and settlement cost of the incident. The more extensively pursued claims tended to involve more severe injuries, and within each disposition category higher settlement sums were associated with the more severe injuries. There were a number of exceptions, however, such as a number of major injuries and death incidents that were described in claim files but were abandoned or did not result in legal action.

Hospitals and other institutions were named in 39% of the claims, a substantial number of which were warning files. The median payment, when made on behalf of hospitals, was $1,710. More frequently named as defendants were practitioners (59%), the bulk of whom were physicians (49%) rather than dentists (7%). Actions against dentists were settled at an early stage, with a relatively small median payment ($855). In contrast, the median settlement on behalf of physicians was $4,190. Very few allied health workers were named in the claims surveyed.

Certain medical specialties contributed disproportionately to malpractice claims in terms of number, patient exposure, disposition and cost outcome. Disproportionate numbers of malpractice claims were filed against orthopedic surgeons (8.8%), anesthesiologists (7.9%), urologists (2.8%) and obstetrician/gynecologists (8.3%). Pediatricians, psychiatrists and ophthalmologists, on the other hand, were rarely cited as defendants. Among several types of practitioners there was an inverse relationship between frequency of claim and size of settlements. The internist was an infrequent target of claim action (6.9%) but paid the highest median settlement ($8,350). Anesthesiologists, on the other hand, were overrepresented in the claim files but paid the lowest median settlement ($1,920).

The patients described in claim files were a representative cross-section, insofar as it could be determined, of the general population of health care consumers. Their demographic profile, in terms of age, sex, and race was not atypical. In a review of 556 cases (Dietz et al., 1973), the injured persons were in the 21–39 and 40–59 age groups, being rather evenly divided between male and female. Most of the injured persons (65%) were married. It is interesting to note that the severity of the injury in about 40% of the cases was regarded as minor. These injuries included lacerations, bruises, contusions, minor scars, rash, broken caps of teeth, minor allergic reactions, operation-induced infection, misset fractures, failure to diagnose glass in a cut, staphylococcus infection from lack of sensitivity to antibiotics and broken ankles.

Physicians' Attitude Survey

A physicians' attitude survey carried out through a mailed questionnaire by the American Medical Association and the American Osteopathic Association (Pabst, 1973) revealed the following:

Forty-eight percent of the survey respondents reported that they had been involved in (17%) or threatened with (27%) a malpractice suit or had a partner who was sued (4%). The remaining 52% had neither been sued nor threatened with malpractice. The majority of the respondents felt that the malpractice problem was worse than ever before. As to the reasons for malpractice suits, both groups (those touched by malpractice suits and those untouched) placed "poor communication" and "aggressive lawyers" at the top of the list. Other listed causes included "declining public regard for doctors" and "increasing complexity of medical practice." The respondents had 8 choices for "the most effective technique for alleviating the malpractice problem." Both groups of physicians considered laws limiting the grounds for suits or laws reducing the size of judgments as a preferred solution, rather than medical or educational improvements.

Lawyers' Attitude Survey

A survey of lawyers (Dietz et al., 1973) handling malpractice cases indicated that each lawyer was involved with very few such cases on the average. The mean was 4 cases per year for defense lawyers and about 1 case every two years for plaintiff lawyers as a national average among lawyers handling malpractice cases. The vast majority of medical malpractice claims are rejected by the lawyers to whom they are brought. The reasons for rejection included no perceived liability (56% of the cases), no injury suffered (7%), economic reasons (23%) and expiration of statute of limitations (4%). The key criterion for accepting cases was the availability of confirming medical advice or medical testimony. Most lawyers went to physician friends or hired physicians to obtain medical advice.

Consumers' Knowledge of and Attitudes toward Medical Malpractice

Peterson (1973) interviewed a random sample of household heads and spouses. Data were collected during hour-long personal interviews with 1,017 respondents. Some of the findings are as follows:

1. Most people felt that doctor-patient relationships today are not as good as they were 20 years ago, although the technical competence of the doctors was viewed as virtually unchanged.
2. Thirty-five percent of the people felt that doctors were no longer as dedicated to their work as in the past. Even more (54%), however, felt that the average American's dedication to work had declined.
3. Just over two fifths of the respondents reported that they, their spouses or a dependent had had a negative medical care experience. Very few reported more than 3 such incidents.
4. Most of the respondents who had had negative experiences felt that the doctor had been negligent in some way. The most frequently perceived failures involved errors of judgment, of which "failure to diagnose correctly" was most often mentioned.
5. Only 8% of those with negative medical care experiences considered seeking the advice of a lawyer. Of those, less than half actually consulted a lawyer.

Physician-Patient Communication

There are four main areas of common concern relating to patient-physician communication and relationship: (1) physician-patient privilege, (2) in a malpractice action, the defendant-physician's access to plaintiff-patient's prior and subsequent medical records where plaintiff has asserted physician-patient privilege, (3) possible remedies to protect the patient against unauthorized disclosure by physicians of medical secrets outside the courtroom, (4) patient's access to his own medical records.

Physician-patient privilege, unlike that of attorney-client, does not exist as common law. However, most states have enacted statutes protecting confidential communication between physicians and their patients from disclosure. Most of these laws state that a physician or surgeon may not be examined in a legal proceeding as to confidential patient communications. Such laws are susceptible to the interpretation that they apply only at trial, but courts have interpreted them to include discovery proceedings as well. The statutes of several states speak of "disclosure" rather than testimony. The more recently enacted statutes of California and Nevada give the patient "a privilege to refuse to disclose, and prevent others from disclosing confidential information."

Usually "communication" is defined as the information acquired by the doctor while attending a patient that was necessary to enable him to prescribe or act for the patient. In some states, it is interpreted more narrowly and may be limited to oral communication, excluding medical records and information about the patient's condition acquired by other means, such as tests or physical examination.

"Privilege" is more narrowly defined, and many of the privilege statutes are explicitly limited to civil actions. Many of the privilege statutes contain exceptions, the most significant of which is the automatic waiver of the privilege where the party's physical condition is in controversy. Laws requiring the reporting of suspected cases of child abuse also often provide for waiver of the privilege in proceedings concerning such cases.

Recently, several states have enacted special laws relating to psychiatrist-patient or psychologist-client communications. Because of the nature of such communications, these statutes create a more comprehensive privilege, either placing them on the same ground as the attorney-client privilege or providing a blanket exemption from disclosure in both civil and criminal actions with few or no exceptions, the most common exception involving a defendant who raises a defense of insanity. Some statutes extend this psychoprivilege to communications with members of the patient's family or members of group therapy sessions.

Most statutes require that two types of medical problems be reported to the appropriate governmental agency—venereal disease and suspected cases of child abuse. Many statutes also require physicians and hospitals to report tuberculosis and other types of contagious diseases, but the identity of the patient is usually protected from public disclosure.

New statutes permit records to be examined and copied by the patient's authorized attorney, as well as by the patient himself.

The Medical Malpractice Insurance Market

The market for medical malpractice insurance is composed of: (1) insurance carriers who sell or underwrite malpractice insurance (sellers), (2) the hospitals and practitioners who buy malpractice insurance (consumers) and (3) insurance salesmen, agents or brokers who sell malpractice insurance (intermediaries).

The malpractice insurance market is more and more specialized and requires increasing knowledge, information and sophistication in order for a carrier to operate with a reasonable probability of earning a profit.

During the decade 1960–70, the size of the medical malpractice insurance market, as measured by premium volume (estimated by multiplying the number of insured dentists, physicians and hospitals by the average premium cost for each category), increased over fivefold, from approximately $65 million in 1960 to over $330 million in 1970. Average premium payments by physicians increased sixfold; those by surgeons, tenfold; and those of hospitals, threefold. The increase in premium volume reflects the increase in both the frequency and the severity of malpractice incidents. Today, virtually no medical professional can afford to practice without some form of malpractice insurance, and most find themselves requiring increasingly higher limits in order to be adequately protected.

Group insurance plans sponsored by state hospital associations or medical societies have grown substantially during the past 5–10 years and should continue to grow and thus consolidate the market.

Features of Medical Malpractice Policies

Professional liability policies are normally written with a given dollar limit on each malpractice occurrence for the insured for the policy year. These limits start as low as $5,000 per occurrence and $15,000 aggregate ($5/15,000) and extend to $15 million per occurrence, depending upon the nature of the risk and the ability of the carrier to provide increased limits.

Liability insurance for hospitals covers three primary areas: professional (or malpractice) liability, general liability (such as happenings on the premises) and workmen's compensation and employees' liability. Comprehensive general liability and malpractice liability protection are generally written in a single policy or contract. Coverage usually includes the officers, administrators, members of the Board of Trustees and directors or governors of the hospital. The general liability coverage applies to employees and sometimes to students or volunteer workers. Professional liability covers the professional staff of the hospital and may include technical and support personnel as well.

Practitioner policies are usually written for 1-year periods but may be written for periods of 3–5 years. In those policies that are written for more than 1 year, there is usually a provision for rate increases or rebates based upon the existence of or frequency of malpractice suits and settlements. The majority of the carriers include premises liability in the basic policy. Some carriers offer premises liability as a rider or extension of the basic policy at an additional premium. Employees of the insured are covered in the policy while acting within the scope of their duties. A professional, such as a resident, other physician or dentist, must be specified and a premium assessed in order to have coverage. Coverage for other employees, such as nurses or technicians, may be limited to cases in which they are included in a suit with the insured.

A distinction should be made between policies written on a "claims incurred" and a "claims made" basis. In policies written on a claims incurred basis, the insured is covered for any claims resulting from an incident that occurred or was alleged to have occurred during the policy period, regardless of when the claim is made. The only limiting factors are the statutes of limitations, which vary from state to state. In a policy written on a claim made basis, the insured is covered for any claim made while the policy is in force, i.e., the coverage ceases when the policy lapses. These policies are usually written to exclude claims based on incidents that occurred prior to the effective date of the policy.

Policies may be canceled at any time by the insured by mailing or delivering the policy with a statement of cancellation to the carrier or its authorized agents. Carriers may cancel by mailing or delivering to the insured or his agent a notice of cancellation to be effective upon the expiration of a given time period. This time period is usually 10 days; however, some states require at least 30 days' advance notice.

Medical malpractice policies have usually carried a provision that the carrier cannot settle a claim without the consent of the insured. Some carriers have eliminated this provision in group plans, so that either the insured or the peer review committee can consent in order to settle a claim.

Deductibles are offered on medical liability insurance for two reasons. One is to lower the cost of insurance to those who seldom have claims or who have a limited number of small claims. Another is to provide insurance to those physicians and institutions who have had poor claims experience or who practice high-risk specialties.

Malpractice Problems For Nonphysician Health Care Professionals

Professionals, such as chiropractors, clinical psychologists, dentists, optometrists, physical therapists, podiatrists and speech therapists/audiologists, fall into the general category of autonomous health care professionals. Although some of them practice in institutions or otherwise come under the direction of other health care professionals, many, and in some professions most, practice solely under their own authority. Malpractice insurance rates for all these professions, with the exception of psychologists and speech therapists/audiologists, are higher for the self-employed practitioner than for employed practitioners.

Although malpractice is not currently considered a serious problem by clinical psychologists, a trend toward more malpractice claims for larger sums is developing. Malpractice insurance has been available to most psychologists through the American Psychological Association since the mid-1950s. Although no rate increases have occurred in the program since it began, a provision was recently added excluding liability coverage for physical injury inflicted during rage-reduction therapy or treatments that involve physical assaults on the patient. Also, a recent expansion of the program provides liability coverage for alleged negligent analysis of test results.

Nurses in a wide variety of specialties, x-ray technicians, medical technologists, dental hygienists, dieticians, physicians' assistants, medical assistants (secretaries, receptionists, aids and others who work in hospitals and in the offices of autonomous health care practitioners) and operating room technicians constitute a category of health care personnel who generally perform their duties under the supervision of a physician or dentist. Most are employees rather than self-employed practitioners. Because they are employed and supervised, malpractice actions arising out of their alleged negligence often fall under the "respondent superior" doctrine, making the employer liable for the negligence of the employee. A sizable portion of the malpractice suits and claims against hospitals stem from the alleged negligence of supervised health care personnel. This doctrine, however, does not abolish the individual liability of the supervised employee who may be named in a malpractice suit in his own right. If his employer's insurance does not provide for his protection, the employee may be forced to absorb the cost of legal fees to defend himself.

Professional liability insurance is available to allied health professionals through various sources, often through special programs sponsored or endorsed by their professional associations.

Recommendations: What to Do and What Not to Do

FOR HOSPITALS.—Hospital administrators contend with the same kind of problems that plague the top management of other large organizations. One of their most difficult problems is the remoteness and alienating aspect of hospitals as perceived by patients. In an effort to manage effectively, hospital management often overlooks the fact that "while hospital routine may be commonplace to hospital personnel, it is strange and mysterious to outsiders." Regulations concerning visitors, mealtimes, treatment procedures and other factors often cause irritation and anxiety. Also, most people enter hospitals fearing the events to follow, and this fact combined with the rising cost of a hospital stay puts the patient in a negative frame of mind.

A number of hospitals have sought to improve patient care by designating an official, or office, to respond to patients' problems or complaints and, in effect, act as a patient advocate or ombudsman. Some mechanism to handle patient grievances must be developed by each hospital. The concept of "patient grievance mechanism" is not generally understood or accepted. Clearly enunciated objectives for such systems should be promulgated, and a number of alternative systems need to be studied to provide some basis for future planning.

FOR PHYSICIANS.—The Interdepartmental Committee on Medical Malpractice of the Armed Forces, set up by the Department of Health, Education, and Welfare (Welch, 1973), made the following recommendations for individual physicians:

1. Physicians should take the time to establish good rapport with their patients, particularly to help them understand the nature of any surgical procedures to be performed and the possible results of these and other procedures.
2. Physicians should be required to attend continuing education courses in their fields. The courses should emphasize new methodology and injury prevention and should be offered at government expense and on government time.
3. Physicians, particularly surgeons, should seek consultation whenever they have the slightest doubt about the correctness of their diagnosis or proposed treatment.
4. Since the facilities and medical specialists at various health care centers vary greatly, patients should be transferred as promptly as possible to centers where they can receive adequate care if facilities or personnel at the center where they were first admitted are inadequate for their medical needs.

5. A uniform record-keeping system to record circumstances surrounding such incidents as slips and falls, suicides and drug-related injuries should be established to provide feedback useful in preventing future injuries of a similar nature.

6. Hospital injury-prevention programs with full-time safety officers responsible for making employees aware of hazards and removing unsafe or inadequate equipment should be established throughout the health care realm.

7. Complete, accurate, legible medical records must be kept on each patient. To facilitate this task, computerized record-keeping systems should be established.

8. Informed consent of patients for surgical or other procedures should be noted, especially on medical records.

9. Health care personnel should be required to attend seminars orienting them to their medical-legal responsibilities and to the practices of their hospitals in handling medical malpractice claims.

REFERENCES

Department of Health, Education, and Welfare: Report of the Secretary's Commission on Medical Malpractice (Washington, D.C.: Government Printing Office, 1973).

Dietz, S. K., Baird, C. B., and Berul, L.: The medical malpractice legal system, in Report of the Secretary's Commission on Medical Malpractice (Washington, D.C.: Government Printing Office, 1973), pp. 87–167.

Pabst, W. R.: A medical opinion survey of physicians' attitude on medical malpractice, in Appendix to Report of the Secretary's Commission on Medical Malpractice (Washington, D.C.: Government Printing Office, 1973), pp. 83–86.

Peterson, J. L.: Consumers' knowledge of and attitudes towards medical malpractice, in Report of the Secretary's Commission on Medical Malpractice (Washington, D.C.: Government Printing Office, 1973), pp. 658–757.

Welch, R., and Shear, B. W.: Malpractice claims in the federal sector, in Report of the Secretary's Commission on Medical Malpractice (Washington, D.C.: Government Printing Office, 1973), pp. 26–37.

Index

T

U

V

X